Carl Auer Systeme

To the Heart
of the Matter

· · · · · · · · · · · · · · ·

Bert Hellinger

Brief Therapies

Translated by Coleen Beaumont

2003

Published by Carl-Auer-Systeme Verlag: **www.carl-auer.de**
Please order our catalogue:
Carl-Auer-Systeme Verlag
Weberstrasse 2
69120 Heidelberg
Germany

Cover: WSP Design, Heidelberg
Coverpainting: "Buchenhain" by Gustav Klimt, 1902
Printed by Koninklijke Wöhrmann B. V., Zutphen
Printed in The Netherlands

ISBN 3-89670-396-X

Title of the original edition:
„Mitte und Maß. Kurztherapien"
© 1999 by Carl-Auer-Systeme Verlag, Heidelberg

Bibliographic information published by Die Deutsche Bibliothek
Die Deutsche Bibliothek lists this publication in the Deutsche Nationalbibliografie;
detailed bibliographic data is available in the Internet at http://dnb.ddb.de.

The wise man said:

What is widely scattered reaches wholeness only
through finding its center
and being collected.
*It is only from the center that abundance has essence
and truth*
and the confusion finds clarity,
simplicity,
as a quiet strength radiating outward,
holding from beneath,
near to the heart of support.

To experience the fullness,
to participate in it,
each of the particulars needn't be known,
spoken,
captured,
performed.

To enter the city, you need only
step through the single gate.
One strike of a bell
sounds many harmonics.
Plucking a ripe apple
requires no knowledge of its origin;
you need only take it in your hand
and eat.

Contents

Introduction

Brief therapies are distinctive in that they concentrate on the heart of the matter, out of the abundance of all the particulars. They move immediately to the center, to the root, to the heart.

Family constellations are also brief therapies because a few steps bring out the previously hidden dynamics in a family, and often, a resolution appears spontaneously. A family constellation lasts 20 to 50 minutes as a rule. This is extremely short when considering how much emerges and how far-reaching the effects may be. Still, the entire family is brought into the picture and many people may be affected in the resolution.

The brief therapies documented in this book, however, concentrate primarily on the individual. The individual is, of course, seen in the context of relationships and connections, but the focus is on one person, in a relationship with one, or perhaps two others. The interest is in resolution or in the restoration of a previously interrupted movement towards another. It may have to do with bringing a feared and avoided truth into awareness by allowing the client to look directly and immediately at the actual situation, and allow this truth to present a resolution. These brief therapies normally last no longer than 15 minutes.

Elements from family constellations also appear in these short therapies, but are then highly concentrated family constellations, reduced to the absolute essentials. They seldom involve more than two or three representatives. At times, the process of resolution takes place with almost no intervention by the therapist, where the client and the representatives operate within a field of energy that reveals a clear direction.

The 63 brief therapies documented here have been extracted from 16 different courses. All these courses for couples or for the seriously ill were recorded on video. In this way, it has been possible to transcribe the exact words that were spoken, and describe movements and gestures where necessary for understanding. As a literal, word-for-word translation is often misleading or difficult to understand, every attempt has been made in the English edition of this book to relay the meaning of the words.

Basically, these short therapies are also short stories, sometimes disturbing, sometimes uplifting, full of drama, or quiet and deep. What they all have in common is that the resolution comes directly from the actual experience, so that each differs from all the others, each is unique.

The order of presentation is chronological, from the various courses, and I have sometimes added additional commentary between stories. The final chapter includes some of the important elements which may lead to resolution.

This book contains my experiences and meetings with many people. I have presented them without any theories, but rather, simply the stories of what happened between us. These encounters have been challenging and enriching for me, and I thank all these people with love and respect.

Bert Hellinger

Acknowledgements

Above all, my appreciation goes to the people I was privileged to meet in these therapeutic encounters.

I would also like to thank the many friends who have helped me in the organization of courses, video recording, and transcribing, which has made this documentation possible. Two in particular deserve special thanks: Johannes Neuhauser and Harald Hohnen.

Thanks to Sylvia GómezPedra, Norbert Linz, and Gunthard Weber for their valuable input.

In friendship
Bert Hellinger

THE WARM HAND OF DEATH
Systemic sclerosis

HELLINGER *to Leah* What is your issue?

LEAH I've had systemic sclerosis for five years, with lung and heart complications.

HELLINGER Could you explain what that is?

LEAH It's a disease of the connective tissues of the body and it also affects the blood vessels.

HELLINGER What are your symptoms?

LEAH The disease has the effect of completely hardening the skin, and also the lungs. That's treated with cortisone, which I've taken for five years. Before the onset of the disease, I suffered from depression and migraines.

HELLINGER That's gone now?

LEAH That got better with the onset of the disease, yes.

HELLINGER I'll do a two-person constellation with you, just you and death.

Leah nods.

HELLINGER Who could be death? Is it a man or a woman?

LEAH A man.

HELLINGER Are you sure? Check it out carefully inside yourself.

LEAH A woman.

HELLINGER I've heard it said that the Vietnamese, during their long civil war, were absolutely fearless regarding death, and said that death was a lady. The inner image of death is often female.

To Leah Choose a representative for yourself and someone to represent death, and place them in relationship to each other.

Leah places the representatives for herself and for death close together, facing one another. They look steadily into each other's eyes.

HELLINGER *after a short while, to Leah's representative* How are you feeling?

LEAH'S REPRESENTATIVE I'm very warm, pleasantly warm. I feel the breath of death. Yes.

DEATH My hands are very warm and tingly.

HELLINGER *to the representative of death* Take her by the hand, with both your hands.

Death reaches out to Leah's representative with both hands. They continue looking steadily into each other's eyes.

HELLINGER *after a while, to Leah's representative* Now, bow your head slightly. A bit deeper. That's it.

She bows her head and remains in that position.

HELLINGER *after a long pause, to Leah* Is that okay for you?

Leah is very moved and nods her head in agreement.

HELLINGER *to Edith, who is in a wheelchair and obviously very ill* I'll work with you now, shall I?

EDITH Do you think anything good will come of it?

HELLINGER If your soul participates, then some good will come of it. My soul will participate as well. Agreed? What are you suffering from?

EDITH Myotrophic lateral sclerosis, including my tongue. What else should I say?

HELLINGER Is this condition curable or not?

EDITH I don't know. I can only eat through a straw.

HELLINGER What do the doctors have to say? What's the prognosis?

EDITH'S DOCTOR The patient had an operation in August for cancer of the bladder and is still under treatment in a clinic. I don't know the prognosis. She was referred to me from another doctor.

HELLINGER I sense that you are afraid to look at this directly.

To another doctor Are you courageous enough to say what the prognosis would be, normally?

DOCTOR I think I have the courage to say what I think, but I want to make it very clear that I don't really know, either. I can only talk about the statistics, and in relation to this neurological degenerative disease, I'm not informed well enough to say. I think that it's the case that what has already been destroyed can't be healed, but that functions may be recovered.

HELLINGER *to Edith* How much time do you give yourself?

EDITH I don't know if this disease is fatal. Is it?

HELLINGER Just according to your inner feelings. How much longer will you live?

EDITH I haven't given that any thought.

HELLINGER Ask the depths of your soul. What does your soul have to say?

EDITH It is silent. *She laughs.* It says that for the others it would be better.

HELLINGER For the others it would be better?

To group I have an image that she does not have long to live. That's the image I have, and I take that seriously. I'll do a constellation that she can simply look at.

To Edith Okay? *Edith nods.*

Hellinger chooses a woman to represent Edith and another woman to represent death. The two representatives spontaneously place themselves facing each other.

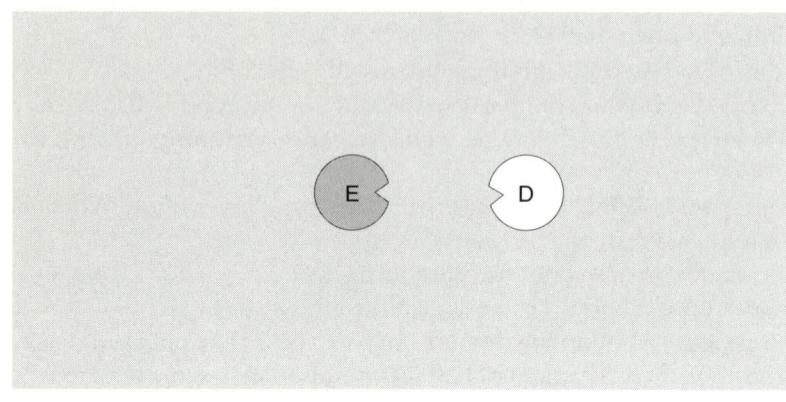

E   Edith's representative
D   Death

After a while, Death steps forward and reaches out a hand to Edith's representative. She leans back somewhat and bows her head to the left. Then, she straightens up again. Death reaches out a bit further. Edith's representative bows slightly forward.

Death moves closer to her and lays a hand on her shoulder. Edith's representative is looking at the floor, and reaches out her left hand. Death takes the hand in both her hands.

Edith's representative covers her eyes with her right arm and turns to the left. She moves backwards towards death. Death puts her arm around her and rests her head behind the woman's head. Death puts her left hand on the back of the woman's head and looks off in the same direction as her.

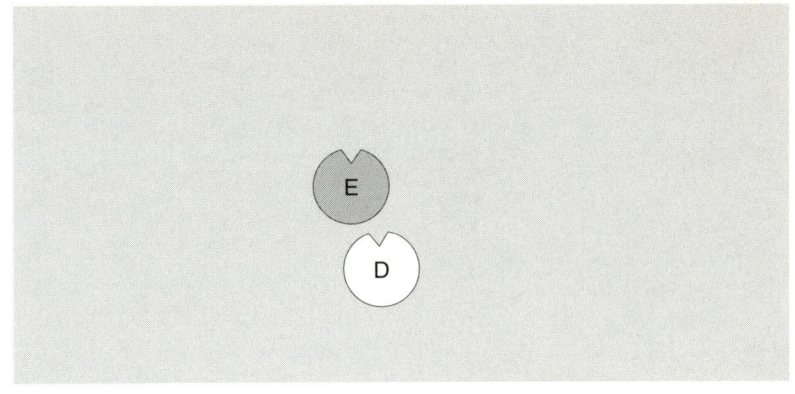

HELLINGER *to Edith's representative* Look Death in the eye and say, "I'm coming."

Edith's representative turns to look at death and takes a step back. They hold hands and look at each other.

EDITH'S REPRESENTATIVE I'm coming.

Death lays her hand on the woman's and holds her right hand. Edith's representative moves towards death and lays her head on her shoulder, but turns away to the left. She then takes a step back. Death continues holding her right hand.

HELLINGER *to Edith's representative* Move in closer once more.

Edith's representative moves close to death again, but again looks off to the left.

HELLINGER *to Edith* There's someone standing in front of your representative. Who is that standing in front of her?

EDITH *(sobs loudly)* My husband. My husband.
HELLINGER Your husband? What about him?
EDITH He's standing there and won't let me go.

Hellinger places a representative for Edith's husband in view of Edith's representative.

19

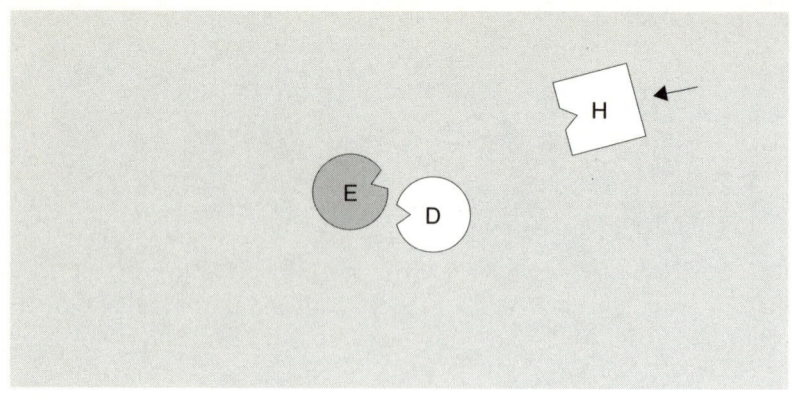

H Husband

HELLINGER *to husband's representative* Just remain standing there.

Edith's representative looks at her husband for a long time.

HELLINGER *to death, as this representative also looks towards the husband* You remain turned towards her.

Hellinger puts Edith's representative's left arm around death. She lays her head on death's shoulder.

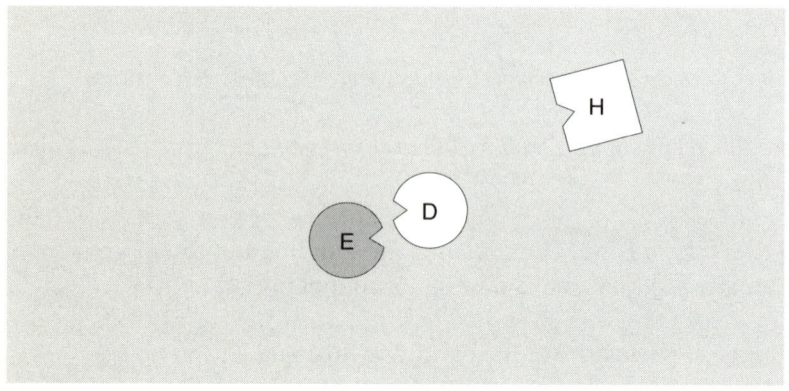

HELLINGER *after a pause* Okay, that was it.

Hellinger *to group* A therapist who's afraid of death can't help. You can't help if you're afraid to look death in the eye.

There's an exercise that I do for myself when there's a client with a life or death issue and I don't know what to do. I imagine the client's death standing some distance from me, and I wait for a signal. Sometimes a signal comes and I can help the client. In that way, I'm in harmony with death.

To a participant who makes an objection Look at the client first, that's important. Often we feel some resistance, and it seems to be justified. When I feel that, I look carefully at the client and test it out. I ask if this will help and nourish, if it will make the person stronger or if it will make them weaker.

Participant Ask the patient right now.
Hellinger No. You can't do that now.
Participant Why not?
Hellinger I would be using her for the satisfaction of the audience. You can't do that. You have to exercise extreme caution.

To a participant who wants to raise another question in this direction I don't want to let myself get drawn into this. Those are questions for someone who thinks they can control the results. I don't have any control over the results, I just bring something out and trust whatever emerges. I trust that there will be an effect without me getting in the middle. I can't step between her soul and what has happened, and such questions would do just that. It seems, on the one hand, that I'm doing something quite presumptuous. On the other hand, it is full of humility, because it leaves things up to the client and trusts that she'll find the right path. It's not what just happened here that supplies the right answer, it simply sets something in motion and opens up a way.

Later

Hellinger *to Edith, an hour later as he sees her laughing* You're laughing!
Edith In fact, I like to laugh.

HELLINGER *to a participant who asks if it isn't presumptuous and danger-ous to speak about death, as he did earlier with Edith* It would be fright-ening if I thought that. We could also ask what others were aware of. Were they aware of something different than I was, or did they pre-fer not to be aware of what came into their consciousness?

You can see immediately if you're in harmony with what's hap-pening or not. Edith was completely in harmony with what hap-pened, and she just told me that she's feeling better. What is true is that the patient herself has no fear. It's others who are afraid. The patient herself knows what's going on with her and can look at it directly.

PARTICIPANT It also seems dangerous to me what you're doing here – this way of treating death and the seriousness of life.

HELLINGER It is dangerous. It pushes to the outer limits and requires the utmost courage from the therapist. It's easier to pull back and hide behind conditionals. The patient is then betrayed and can't take a stand. When I speak to the issue this clearly, there's no room for playing around and it comes to the absolute gravity at the heart of the matter. Then the patient is completely with herself, and she'll also defy me at the moment when the heart of things is reached. Up to that point, it's a different story. She won't trust me if I hide.

I present my awareness as if it had absolute validity in that moment when I say it. Actually, I can't see anything else at that moment. But I'm not alone. The patient has her awareness and so do those in the group. When the patient or others have a different awareness, then that is also included. That's why I'm not worried that something could go wrong.

ANOTHER PARTICIPANT I have to ask how you can be so certain.

HELLINGER If I forget something important or if the work just doesn't move on and we have to break it off, I have often noticed that later something emerges for the client, or for someone near to them, that allows the work to continue. I trust others as well. I join my soul with the patient's soul, but at the same time I have a sense of a greater soul that encompasses everything and that works invisibly. With courage, I can allow that to work.

In Carlos Castaneda's books about Don Juan, the Shaman, there's something about the enemies of knowledge. The primary foe is fear. Whoever is afraid cannot become aware. Clarity only comes to those who have overcome their fear.

"THERE IS NOTHING THAT IS MORE THAN YOUR MOTHER"
Trigeminal pain, migraines, anxieties

HELLINGER What's your difficulty?

ANNA I feel energy fields, I have trigeminal pain, migraines, various allergic reactions, and anxieties.

HELLINGER That's a whole lot. Are you married?

ANNA Married but recently separated.

HELLINGER Have you got children?

ANNA No.

HELLINGER Why did you separate?

ANNA We just drifted apart, and as my reactions to the radiation therapy got worse, my husband said I should find myself a place of my own.

HELLINGER And you can understand that? You appear happy with the separation. Looking at your face, it's a relief for you.

ANNA Partly.

HELLINGER Partly is enough.

To group Could you see how happy she looked about the separation? Okay. What happened in your family of origin?

ANNA I was a premature baby.

HELLINGER How premature?

ANNA I was born in the eight month.

HELLINGER Were you in an incubator?

ANNA *crying* I was immediately taken from my mother and moved to another hospital.

HELLINGER To another hospital?

ANNA *crying* My mother didn't see me for a while.

HELLINGER For how long?

ANNA I don't know exactly, perhaps a month.

HELLINGER Did your mother suffer problems during the birth?

ANNA She almost bled to death. She told me that the placenta didn't come out, so the doctors pressed on her belly and she nearly bled to death. Then there was an outbreak of some infection in the hospital, so they put her in a huge hall all alone and she felt very lonely.

HELLINGER This is a traumatic event, not a systemic one. What should we do with you now?

24

ANNA I don't know.
HELLINGER Shall I do something?
ANNA Yes.
HELLINGER Then I'll do a peculiar exercise with you, shall I?
ANNA What is it?
HELLINGER You'll see. But, it's nothing that will embarrass you. Okay?
ANNA Okay.

Hellinger chooses a representative for her mother and has her lie on her back on the floor. He has Anna lie next to her with her head at the same level.

HELLINGER *to the mother* All you have to do is look up. Otherwise you don't have to do anything except be there.
To Anna Turn your head towards her and look at her with love.

After a short time, as he sees that Anna is very touched Breathe deeply.
After a while What did you call your mother when you were a child?
ANNA Mommy.
HELLINGER Look at her and say, "Mommy."
ANNA Mommy.
HELLINGER Breathe deeply. Breathe into your belly, and look at her. "Mommy."
ANNA Mommy.
HELLINGER "Dear Mommy." Keep looking at her as you speak.
ANNA Dear Mommy.
HELLINGER Say, "I take this from you."
ANNA I take this from you.
HELLINGER "Even at the price you had to pay."

Anna weeps.

HELLINGER Look at her. Look at her and say, "Even at the price you had to pay." You have to look at her.
ANNA Even at the price you had to pay.
HELLINGER "Dear Mommy."
ANNA Dear Mommy.
HELLINGER *after a while* How do you feel saying that?
ANNA I can't say.
HELLINGER Do you really take it?

ANNA I don't know.

HELLINGER How is your mother doing?

ANNA My mother? I always have the feeling she doesn't take me in, or she doesn't let me go.

HELLINGER So far I've only seen that you don't take her in. Look at her! Say, "Dear Mommy."

ANNA *speaking through suppressed crying* Dear Mommy.

HELLINGER "I take you as my mother."

ANNA I take you as my mother.

HELLINGER "And you may have me as your child."

ANNA And you may have me as your child.

HELLINGER "I will always stay with you."

ANNA I will always stay with you.

HELLINGER "Dear Mommy."

ANNA Dear Mommy.

HELLINGER Say it calmly in a normal voice. "Dear Mommy."

ANNA Dear Mommy.

HELLINGER "I take you as my mother."

ANNA I take you as my mother.

HELLINGER "And you may have me as your child."

ANNA And you may have me as your child.

HELLINGER "I'll always stay with you."

ANNA I'll always stay with you.

HELLINGER How is that?

ANNA Good.

HELLINGER Okay, that was it.

To the representative of the mother Thank you for participating.

To Anna, as she sits next to him I have a suspicion about the energy fields. They're nothing but your mother.

ANNA My mother?

HELLINGER They are nothing but your mother. Is that a pleasant thought?

ANNA I've always had the feeling I was losing energy.

HELLINGER What did I say?

ANNA The energy field is my mother.

HELLINGER Exactly.

ANNA And that which is positive.

HELLINGER Exactly.

ANNA What more could there be? *She laughs.*

HELLINGER I'll tell you a secret. There is nothing that is more than your mother. Agreed?

Anna laughs and nods.

HELLINGER For the therapists I would like to explain something about this method. Often when there is a separation, there is an identification. Anna suffers with her mother. What her mother suffered, she suffers as well. If you have the two lie down together and ask the daughter to look at her mother with love, the identification can be dissolved. As soon as love flows, the identification dissolves. It's only possible to have an identification when there is no one there, because in an identification I merge with the other person. As soon as there is actually a separate person there who can be seen, so that the love can flow, the identification is dissolved.

"Buy a VW Fox"
Fear of auto accidents

HELLINGER What's with you?

ILSE I'm terrified I'm going to have a car accident.

HELLINGER Have you ever had an accident?

ILSE Not yet, I haven't ever had a car accident.

HELLINGER I once had an engineer in a course who bought a Mercedes. In his family, that wasn't permissible. One day he was driving down the freeway and suddenly someone ran into him from behind. Then he could breathe more easily! He had paid for his Mercedes.

ILSE I bought myself a car that my husband didn't want me to buy.

HELLINGER How long have you had it?

ILSE Three years.

HELLINGER What kind of car?

ILSE A BMW. *Laughter in the group.*

HELLINGER And what does your husband drive?

ILSE A VW Golf.

HELLINGER I'll give you a suggestion. Buy a VW Fox!

ILSE That's what I used to have. *Laughter in the group.*

"I'm the right one for you"
Mother of a severely handicapped child

HELLINGER *to Katharina* What is it?

KATHARINA I have a compulsive neurosis and depression.

HELLINGER What do you do compulsively?

KATHARINA I take many precautions. For myself it's not as important as it is for my handicapped son who lives in another city. When I drive up there, I take many precautions. I wash myself and every item I take with me.

HELLINGER So you have a handicapped son.

KATHARINA Yes.

HELLINGER What kind of handicap does he have?

KATHARINA He's 100 percent mentally and physically handicapped.

HELLINGER What about your husband?

KATHARINA He died three years ago.

HELLINGER What happened that your son is so severely handicapped?

KATHARINA He's been like that since birth. At that time they looked for the cause, but nothing concrete could be found.

HELLINGER How did you react, as parents?

KATHARINA My husband was very calm about it, but I ran from doctor to doctor. We also went to Berlin to Charité, and everywhere.

HELLINGER Did either of you have feelings of guilt about the disabilities, you or your husband?

KATHARINA I asked myself what I had done wrong, but I couldn't come up with anything.

HELLINGER How old were you when your child was born?

KATHARINA Twenty-eight.

Hellinger chooses a representative for the handicapped son and places him facing his mother.

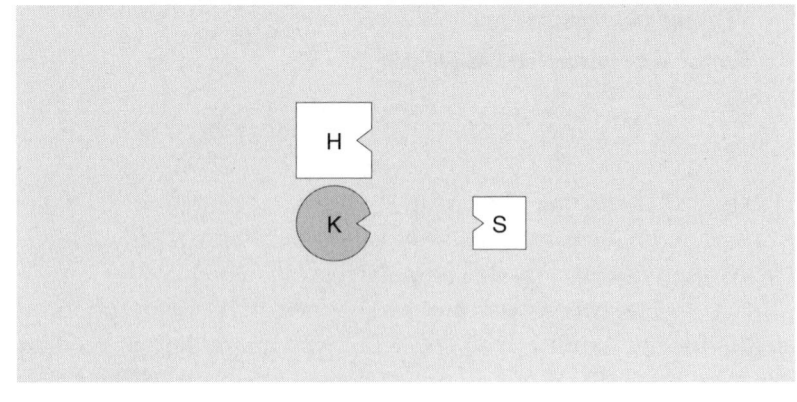

K   **Katharina**
S   Son, physically and mentally handicapped
H   Hellinger

HELLINGER *to Katharina* Put your arm around me and look at your son. Tell him, "I take you as my child."
KATHARINA I take you as my child.
HELLINGER "In my heart."
KATHARINA In my heart.
HELLINGER "And in my arms."
KATHARINA And in my arms.
HELLINGER "I'll care for you as best I can."
KATHARINA I'll care for you as best I can.
HELLINGER "And I entrust you to a greater power."
KATHARINA And I entrust you to a greater power.
HELLINGER "And I place myself within this power."
KATHARINA And I place myself within this power.
HELLINGER "To which I entrust you."
KATHARINA To which I entrust you.
HELLINGER Go to your son and touch him with both hands.

Hellinger leads her to her son. She puts her hand on his arms and strokes him.

30

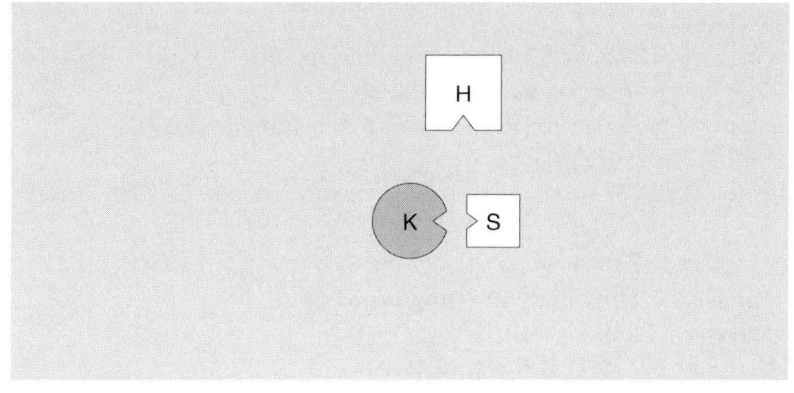

HELLINGER Touch him in a healing way, with both hands. In a healing way with both hands. Begin with his head, firmly, so he can feel you touching him.

She strokes him firmly with both hands, beginning with his head, moving over his cheeks and down his shoulders and arms.

HELLINGER Look into his eyes and say, "I am the right one for you."
KATHARINA *continuing to hold and stroke him* I am the right one for you.
HELLINGER "I am your mother."
KATHARINA I am your mother. I am the right one for you. I am your mother.
To Hellinger as she releases her son Could I say something else? I used to avoid driving up to see him very often because of all the precautions I felt compelled to take. Now, I go more often and do whatever I feel is the right thing to do. Every time I go, I have to overcome this, but when I'm there, I take him in my arms and hug him.

She is very moved.

HELLINGER Exactly. Do exactly that.

She holds her son again with both hands.

HELLINGER Tell him, "No one is better for you than me, your mother."
KATHARINA *in tears* No one is better for you than me, your mother.
HELLINGER How is the son doing?

31

SON Good.

To his mother Above all, when you hold me firmly. I didn't feel good when you let me go just then for a while.

HELLINGER *to Katharina* Right, you have healing hands.

The son moves to his mother and they embrace tenderly for a long time.

HELLINGER *to Katharina, as they release their embrace* Look at him.

After a while How are you doing now?

KATHARINA Fine.

HELLINGER I'll leave it there, okay?

KATHARINA Yes.

"I LET YOU GO WITH LOVE"
Anxiety and depression

HELLINGER *to Carole* What's your issue?
CAROLE I have a dead twin sister and I suffer from anxiety and depression.
HELLINGER When did your twin sister die?
CAROLE At the age of one year and fifteen days.
HELLINGER Who is the elder of the two of you?
CAROLE I am.
HELLINGER We'll set up a constellation with two people, you and your twin sister.

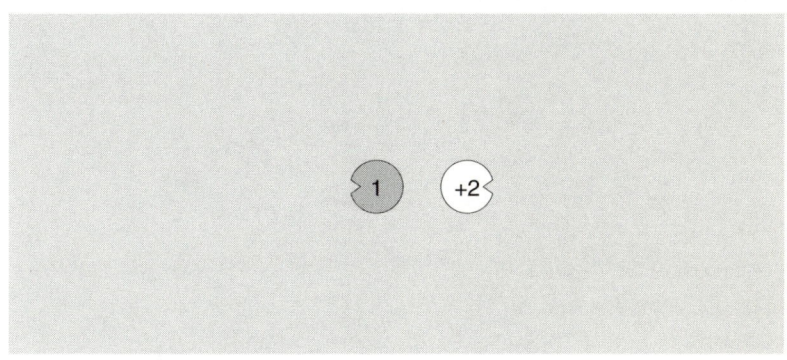

1   **First-born twin sister (Carole)**
2   Second-born twin sister, who died at the age of one

HELLINGER *to the representative of Carole* How do you feel?
FIRST-BORN TWIN I feel a shooting pain in my lungs and in my heart. I feel very much alone and I feel anxious. I don't know what's behind me. I can feel something, but I don't know what.
HELLINGER *to deceased twin* How are you feeling?
SECOND-BORN TWIN I also feel alone, but light. I don't feel any connection to anything behind me, so it's a bit like floating. *She laughs.* But good. I feel fine, too.
HELLINGER *to group* Death holds nothing terrible for a child …
To Carole … if she is released, if she is let go. In the Duino Elegies, Rilke said of those who passed on early that it makes it difficult for

33

them when we grieve for them excessively. Their light movements are hampered by our grief. You could see that light movement here. Take your place in the constellation.

Carole replaces her representative in the constellation.

HELLINGER *as she is in her place* How is that for you?
CAROLE Something's pulling me down.

Hellinger places her to the side where she can see her twin sister.

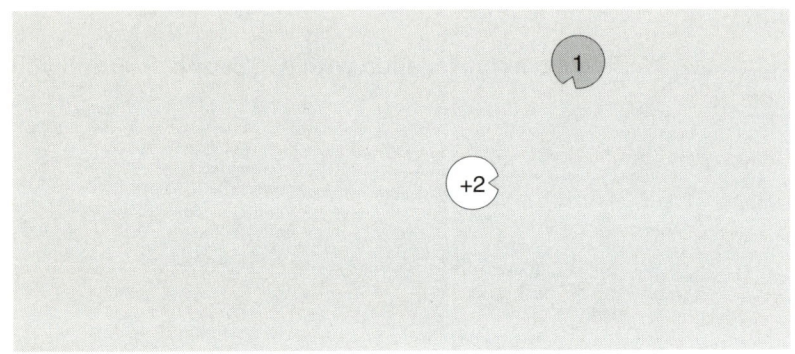

HELLINGER How's that?
CAROLE I can see her.
HELLINGER *to the deceased sister* How do you feel?
SECOND-BORN TWIN The same. I feel fine.
HELLINGER *to Carole* Look at her.
To deceased sister You don't have to look over here. Look in your own direction.
To Carole Tell her, "I let you go, with love."
CAROLE I let you go, with love.
HELLINGER "And after a while, I'll come, too."
CAROLE And after a while, I'll come, too.
HELLINGER How's that?
CAROLE So strange.
HELLINGER Stand behind her.

34

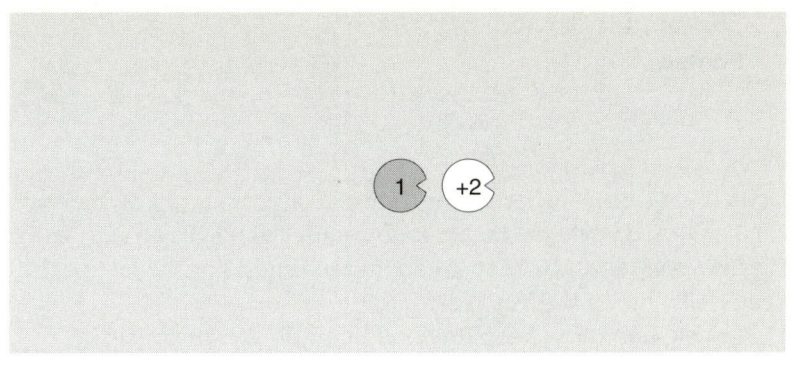

HELLINGER How is that?
CAROLE I'm falling backwards.
HELLINGER Move back.

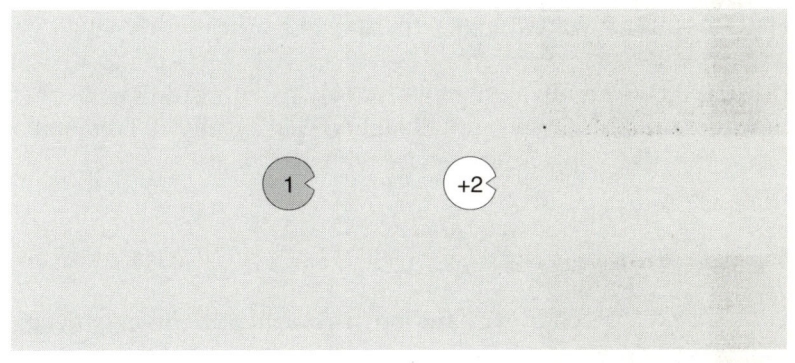

HELLINGER How is it now?
CAROLE That's good.
HELLINGER Say it once more, "I let you go, with love."
CAROLE I let you go with love.
HELLINGER "And after a while, I'll come, too."
CAROLE And after a while, I'll come, too. *She breathes out audibly.*
HELLINGER How is that?
CAROLE It's fine.
HELLINGER How is it for the twin sister?
SECOND-BORN TWIN Good. That feels good. It's a bit of a pleasant feeling. I feel a deep love for her, and I'm happy that she'll come later.
HELLINGER *to Carole* Okay, that's it.

"Mommy, I'll hold you"
Diarrhea

DORA I have been suffering for a couple of years in that whenever I eat, I have to dash to the toilet for hours afterwards. It can start within five minutes, and I have to go about ten times. For the last year it's been really bad. I feel very restricted.

HELLINGER Can't you keep the food in, or do you throw up?

DORA No, I have diarrhea. For about the last year, it's been so bad that I don't trust myself to be around other people.

HELLINGER What about your mother?

DORA My mother had a mastectomy four years ago. She had breast cancer. Now she's doing pretty well.

HELLINGER How were things with you and your mother when you were a child?

DORA I can only really remember that my parents didn't have much time for us because they worked nights. That's really all I remember.

HELLINGER We'll do a little exercise with you, okay?

DORA Yes.

Hellinger sits opposite Dora.

HELLINGER Close your eyes and open your mouth. Breathe deeply. Faster.

Hellinger takes her hands and gently bows her head a bit forward. They remain like that for a short while.

HELLINGER What did you call your mother when you were a child?

DORA Mommy.

HELLINGER Say, "Mommy."

DORA Mommy.

HELLINGER "I'll hold you tightly."

DORA I'll hold you tightly.

HELLINGER "Really tightly."

DORA Really tightly.

HELLINGER Breathe deeply and a bit faster. Go with your movement. Give in to your own movement.

Dora lays her head in Hellinger's lap. He puts his arm around her.

HELLINGER Tell her, "I'll hold you tightly."
DORA I'll hold you tightly.
HELLINGER And do that. Tightly. Yes, really tightly.

Dora puts her arms around Hellinger and holds on to him tightly.

HELLINGER "Mommy, I'll hold you tightly."
DORA Mommy, I'll hold you tightly.
HELLINGER "Really tightly."
DORA Really tightly.
HELLINGER "Please stay."
DORA Please stay.
HELLINGER "I'll hold on to you tightly."
DORA I'll hold on to you tightly.
HELLINGER "And please hold me tightly."
DORA And please hold me tightly.

Hellinger has her straighten up and they hold each other tightly in an embrace.

HELLINGER "I'll hold you tightly, and please, you hold me tightly."
DORA I'll hold you tightly, and please, you hold me tightly.
HELLINGER "Please, Mommy."
DORA Please, Mommy.
HELLINGER "Mommy, I take you and I hold you tightly."
DORA Mommy, I take you and I hold you tightly.
HELLINGER "Really tightly."
DORA Really tightly.
HELLINGER Breathe deeply. That's it, yes.

After a while Hellinger releases his embrace, but continues to hold Dora's hands. Dora sits facing him and looks at him.

HELLINGER How is that?
DORA Fine.
HELLINGER Yes, exactly. Now you'll gain some weight. Right?
DORA Yes.

"MOTHER, MY HEART BEATS FOR YOU"
Cardiac arrhythmia

URSULA I'm sitting here because I have been suffering from cardiac arrhythmia for the past thirteen years. Sometimes it's worse, sometimes better. I've also had phases when I thought I'd got over it, but it always comes back. What I've noticed is that every time I have the feeling that everything is okay, that everything's going well, I have another attack, usually in the night. I wake up in total panic. I imagine that this has something to do with my family of origin. I lost my father when I was twelve and a half.

HELLINGER What did he die of?

URSULA He died of a heart attack, very suddenly. When I read your book, I talked to my mother about it. I told her that I had always had the feeling that she died at the same time. For years, I was trying to find my mother, and sometimes I feel like I'm still trying.

HELLINGER Imagine that your mother is sitting in front of you. Tell her, "My heart beats for you."

Ursula puts her hands in her lap, and collects herself, looking forward.

URSULA *after a while* Mother, my heart beats for you.

HELLINGER Say it with love.

URSULA Mother, my heart beats for you.

HELLINGER Say it with love.

Ursula sighs, puts her hands to her heart, looks up and nods.

HELLINGER Keep looking straight ahead. You were doing well just now.

Ursula hesitates.

HELLINGER *to group* Now she's moved into thinking. A minute ago she was in touch with the right feelings.

To Ursula Tell her that as a child would.

URSULA Mother, my heart beats for you.

38

HELLINGER "With love." Add that.
URSULA *sighs* Mother, my heart beats for you, with love.

She breathes deeply and nods.

HELLINGER *after a while* Imagine that your father is next to her, both of
them together. Then say, "My heart beats for both of you, with love."
URSULA My heart beats for both of you, with love.

She lets her arms drop to her sides.

HELLINGER Now you have to allow your heart to do it as well. Right?
URSULA *laughs* Absolutely.
HELLINGER Okay, that's all.

"I'LL WAIT A BIT LONGER"
Saying goodbye to a deceased husband

HELLINGER *to Gabrielle* What's going on with you?
GABRIELLE My husband died two and a half years ago.
HELLINGER We'll set up a constellation with two people, you and your husband.

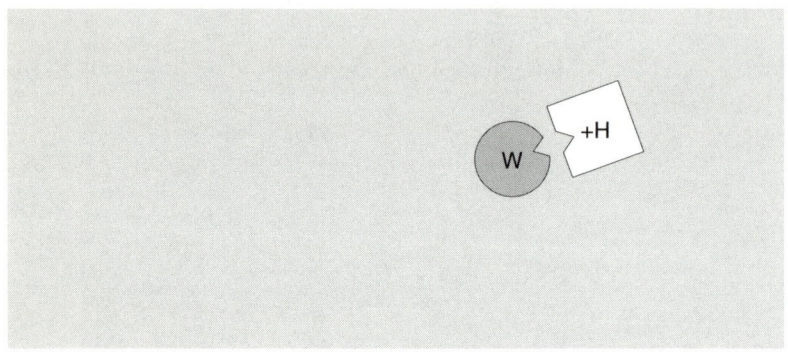

+H   Husband
W   Wife (Gabrielle)

HELLINGER *to husband's representative* How is that for you?
HUSBAND I'm being drawn from something behind me. I have an expansive field around me, and she's inside it.
HELLINGER *to Gabrielle's representative* And for you?
WIFE I feel very agitated, and I have to keep looking into his eyes, almost as if I'm hypnotized.

Hellinger moves the husband and then the wife so that they're further apart.

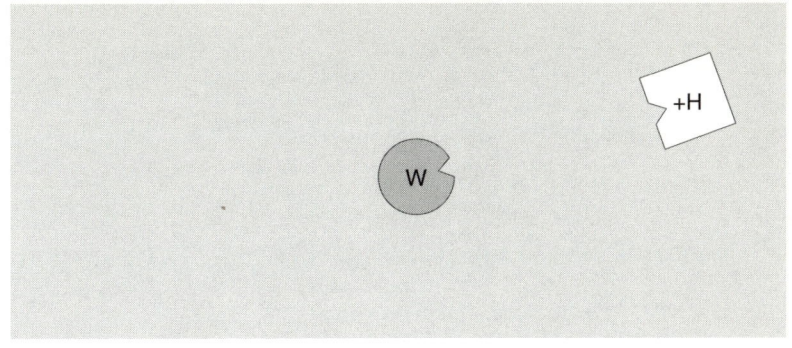

HELLINGER *to husband's representative* How's that?

HUSBAND It's better. Now she's just an ordinary person. But, there's still something in that look, something mesmerizing. That's still there, but it's considerably more comfortable.

HELLINGER *to Gabrielle's representative* And you?

WIFE If it has to be, then it has to be. I like looking at him. I'm less agitated than before, but I'm still hot. It's a pity he wants to get away from me.

HELLINGER Tell him, "I'm still waiting for something."

WIFE I'm still waiting for something.

HELLINGER How does that feel?

WIFE That's hard for me. Actually, I don't want to let him really go yet. I still feel a resistance.

HELLINGER Tell him, "I'll leave you."

WIFE I'll leave you.

HELLINGER "For a little while."

WIFE For a little while.

HELLINGER How is that?

WIFE Better.

HELLINGER Take a couple of steps backwards, wherever you'd like.

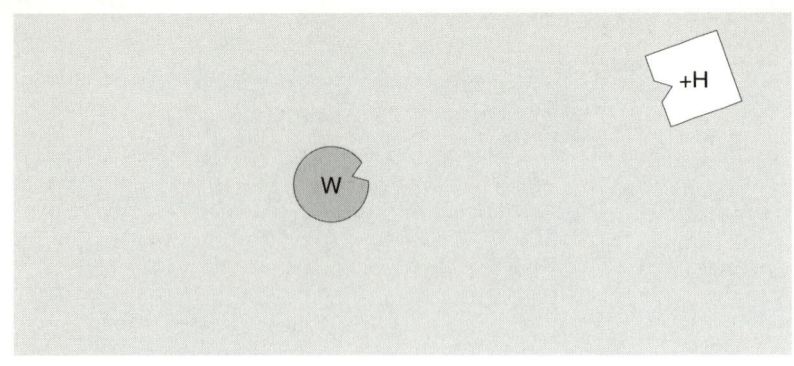

HELLINGER How is it, now?
WIFE That's getting better. I think I could move back slowly.
HELLINGER Move a bit more.

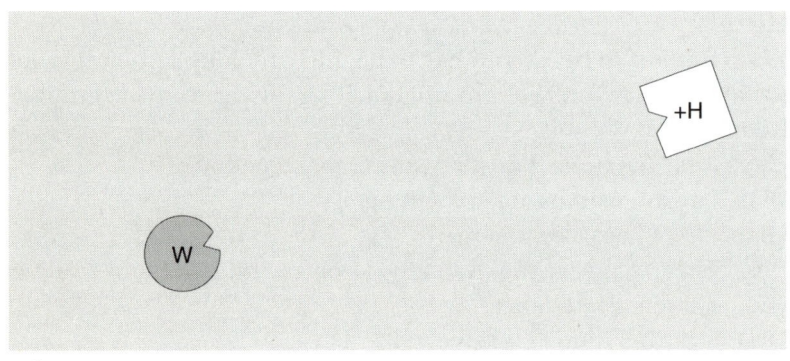

HELLINGER Now, how is it?
WIFE *(laughs)* There's a sentence on the tip of my tongue.
HELLINGER Go ahead and say it.
WIFE Take care of yourself. I'm leaving now. *She laughs.*
HELLINGER *to Gabrielle* Is that okay for you?
GABRIELLE Yes, I think that's best. *She laughs.*
HELLINGER Okay, that's it.

"MAMA, YOU AND I"
Brain hemorrhage

HELLINGER *to Natalie* What's going on with you?

NATALIE I am handicapped as a result of a brain hemorrhage I had eleven years ago. But the acute problem is that for the past six years I've had neurological pains on the right side of my body and they're getting worse. I've tried a lot of different things for this, but I don't seem to be getting anywhere. I just get my hopes up, and then they're dashed. I don't know why.

HELLINGER Are you married?

NATALIE I was married eighteen years ago. It only lasted for three years.

HELLINGER What happened?

NATALIE *(sighs)* Nothing dramatic. It's hard to say, really.

HELLINGER Who wanted the separation?

NATALIE First my husband left me, then later, when he wanted to come back, I wasn't interested anymore.

HELLINGER Did something happen in connection with this brain hemorrhage?

NATALIE Nothing specific happened. I had had a long history of high blood pressure, for about fourteen years.

HELLINGER What do you want from me?

NATALIE I want to get some clue as to what is blocked that keeps me from being able to allow healing influences to touch me.

HELLINGER What happened in your family of origin?

NATALIE My parents had problems pretty early in their marriage. From the time I was about ten, my father had a girlfriend, and when I was about twenty, he separated from my mother.

HELLINGER Which of your parents are you angry with?

NATALIE I used to reject my mother, because she was so clearly difficult. My father was more reserved, and then he disappeared and wasn't an easy target. But something in me has softened in recent years. I mean, I've forgiven my mother for how it was back then, the break up in the family and all the conflict.

Hellinger chooses a woman to represent Natalie's mother and asks her to sit next to Natalie.

43

HELLINGER *to representative of Mother* You just look forward.

To Natalie And you look at her.

NATALIE *(after a while)* She seems so unreachable.

HELLINGER *(after a while)* When you were a child, what did you call your mother?

NATALIE Mama.

HELLINGER Look over at her. Look at her and say, "Mama."

NATALIE *(in a quiet voice)* Mama.

HELLINGER Breathe deeply, with your mouth open, and say, "Mama."

NATALIE Mama.

HELLINGER A bit louder.

NATALIE Mama.

HELLINGER "Please, Mama, please."

NATALIE Mama, please.

HELLINGER "Mama, you and I."

NATALIE Mama, you and I.

HELLINGER *(after a while)* What is it?

NATALIE She's still so far away.

HELLINGER Tell her, "I'll stand by you."

NATALIE I'll stand by you.

HELLINGER "Dear Mama."

NATALIE Dear Mama.

HELLINGER "I'll stand by you."

NATALIE I'll stand by you.

After a while I feel closer, but not like I'd like.

HELLINGER What's harder, the pain or the love for your mother?

NATALIE Both.

HELLINGER Which is more difficult?

NATALIE At first I thought the pain, but I'm not so sure.

HELLINGER The love is more difficult. It hurts more. What could relieve the pain?

NATALIE Love.

HELLINGER Love for?

After a pause, to the mother's representative Put your hand on her shoulder, very gently.

To Natalie Look at her.

After a while How do you feel now?

NATALIE Better.

HELLINGER That's what relieves the pain. Do you see?

44

NATALIE *(strongly)* Yes.

HELLINGER But you've still got a long way to go.

NATALIE The way it is now, I feel the love that comes across, but how do I put that into practice? I don't know how to use that.

HELLINGER Exactly. You've got a long way to go. I'll tell you something about love. It's the most difficult thing. Not having love, but admitting it in. Okay?

NATALIE Yes.

PARTICIPANT I have a question about forgiveness. As the affected one, how can I forgive so that I'm free to experience love and form a relationship? How do I let go of all the old baggage?

HELLINGER Forgiveness has a bad effect. Imagine a child telling her mother, "I forgive you." How would the mother feel?

PARTICIPANT Bad.

HELLINGER Of course. What would be a different solution? The child says, "Mama, you have given me so much." Do you feel the difference?

PARTICIPANT Yes.

Three Siblings – "We take you, with all that entails"
Incurable genetic disease (Huntington's Chorea[1])

HELLINGER *to three siblings* What's the problem with you three?
FIRST CHILD My father suffered from a genetic disease. It's a dominant gene, which means that there's a fifty percent chance that we will also get it.
HELLINGER What disease is it?
FIRST CHILD Huntington's Chorea. It's a disease that normally shows up between the ages of perhaps thirty and fifty.
HELLINGER Have you got children?
FIRST CHILD Yes, two.
HELLINGER Are they in danger of getting the disease?
FIRST CHILD If I get it, then they've got a fifty percent chance of getting it. If I don't get it, then they won't get it either.
HELLINGER I'll tell you a story. There was a woman, once, in a course, who was dressed all in black. I asked her to tell me two stories that moved her, one from her early childhood and one from the present. If you compare the two stories, you can see what is meaningful in her life. The first story, from when she was five years old, was the song

> *Lullaby, and good night,*
> *With roses bedight*
> *And lilies o'erspread*
> *There pillow thy head.*
> *To awake in the morn,*
> *When the day is reborn.*
> *Lullaby, and good night*
> *Angels watch through the night*
> *Lay thee down now and rest*
> *May these hours be blest*
> *Lay thee down now and rest*
> *May these hours be blest.*

1   Huntington's Chorea is an incurable disease which affects half of the offspring of the affected parent. Its onset is in middle age, and is characterized by trembling extremities and a rapid physical and mental deterioration.

The second story, from the present, was "The Black Spider," the movie version. Drug addicts break into a chemical factory and throw some containers around. It releases a cloud of poisonous gas that spreads through the land and destroys all life.

After that, I asked her about her family of origin. She said she had three brothers. The first brother died at the age of three weeks, the second at the age of three months, and the third at the age of three years. She came from a family of hemophiliacs. The first story was a lamentation for her brothers.

She had two sons herself. I asked her about her husband. She said that he stood one hundred percent by her, including her genetic inheritance. Then I asked about her sons and she said that they also stood by her completely.

I suggested that she tell her husband and her children that she regarded their complete support as a gift. She couldn't do that. That was too much for her.

Okay, these stories have told you something.

Hellinger chooses a representative for the father and places the three siblings facing him.

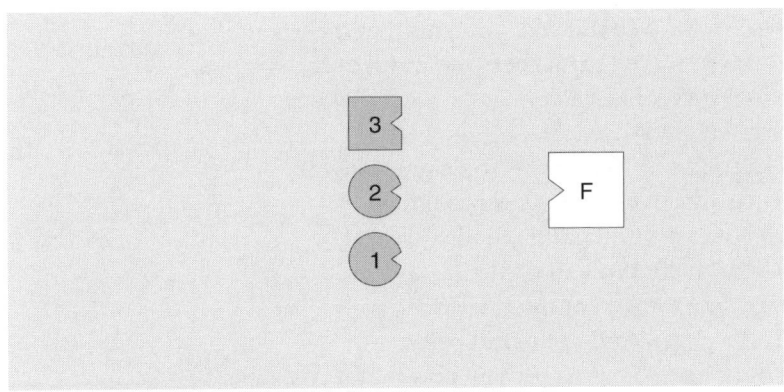

F	Father
1	**First Child, a daughter**
2	**Second Child, a daughter**
3	**Third Child, a son**

HELLINGER *to father's representative* Look at your children. Is there anything you want to say to them?

FATHER I feel a tightness. I don't feel like I can say anything to my children.

HELLINGER *to First child* Tell him, "I take you as my father."

FIRST CHILD I take you as my father.

HELLINGER "With all that entails."

FIRST CHILD With all that entails.

HELLINGER How is that?

FIRST CHILD It's good.

HELLINGER "I take from you, at the full price."

FIRST CHILD I take from you, at the full price.

HELLINGER "That it costs you and me."

FIRST CHILD That it costs you and me.

HELLINGER How is that for the father?

FATHER That's good. I feel somewhat freer, that is, not as apprehensive as before.

HELLINGER *to Second child* You tell him, too, "I take you as my father."

SECOND CHILD I take you as my father.

HELLINGER "With all that entails."

SECOND CHILD With all that entails.

HELLINGER "And I take it at the full price."

SECOND CHILD And I take it at the full price.

HELLINGER "That it cost you and that it costs me."

SECOND CHILD That it cost you and that it costs me.

HELLINGER "Dear Papa."

SECOND CHILD Dear Papa.

HELLINGER *to Third child* You say it as well.

THIRD CHILD I take you as my father.

HELLINGER "With all it entails."

THIRD CHILD With all it entails.

HELLINGER "And at the full price."

THIRD CHILD And at the full price.

HELLINGER "That it cost you and that it costs me."

THIRD CHILD That it cost you and that it costs me.

HELLINGER "Dear Papa."

THIRD CHILD Dear Papa.

HELLINGER Go to your father, all three of you, and embrace him.

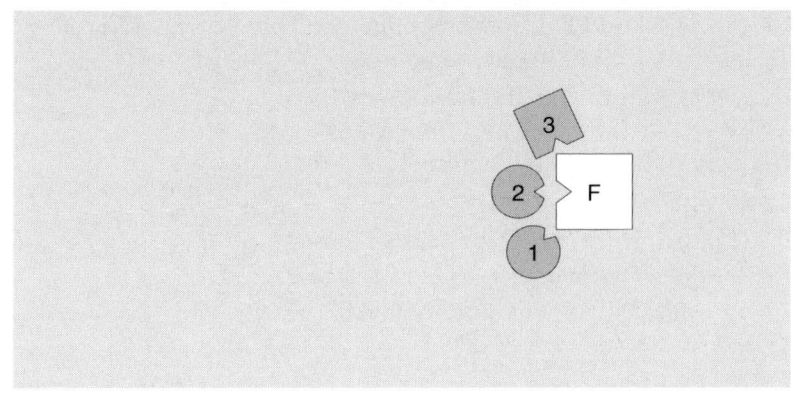

HELLINGER *after a while, as the embrace comes to an end* How is the father feeling?

FATHER Good. Yes, a lot better than before.

FIRST CHILD *(very moved)* I felt good during the whole constellation, right from the beginning.

SECOND CHILD It was right on, but I wanted to get away from my father. There was something else, as if I had to do something for myself, leaving or staying. It was as if I'd already experienced whatever that embrace was. That was my experience.

THIRD CHILD It was difficult, but good.

HELLINGER *to the brother and sisters* Now move back away, far away – even further – and stand next to each other.

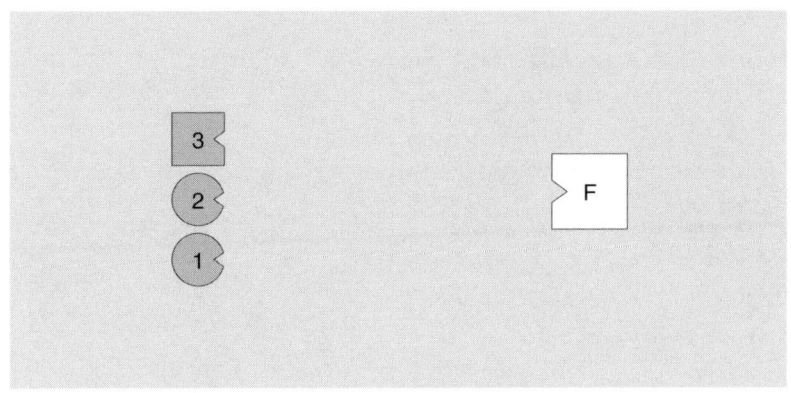

HELLINGER *to Second child* Tell him, "Papa, I'll leave you in peace."

SECOND CHILD Papa, I'll leave you in peace.

HELLINGER "And I'll make something good out of what I have."
SECOND CHILD And I'll make something good out of what I have.
HELLINGER "From you and from Mom."
SECOND CHILD From you and from Mom.
HELLINGER How is that?
SECOND CHILD That's good.
HELLINGER *to Third child* You say that also.
As the representative hesitates Okay, I'll wait.
After a while Do you want to say it, too?
THIRD CHILD Yes.
HELLINGER "Dear Papa."
THIRD CHILD Dear Papa.
HELLINGER "I'll leave you in peace."
THIRD CHILD I'll leave you in peace.
HELLINGER "And I'll make something of what I've got from you."
THIRD CHILD And I'll make something of what I've got from you.
HELLINGER "From you and from Mom."
THIRD CHILD From you and from Mom.
HELLINGER How's that?
THIRD CHILD That's okay.
HELLINGER *to second and third children* You two go and sit down now.

Hellinger brings in the husband of the first daughter, who is present in the group, and places him next to his wife.

HELLINGER *to First child* Have you two got children?
FIRST CHILD Yes, two daughters.

Hellinger chooses two representatives for the daughters and places them to the left of their mother.

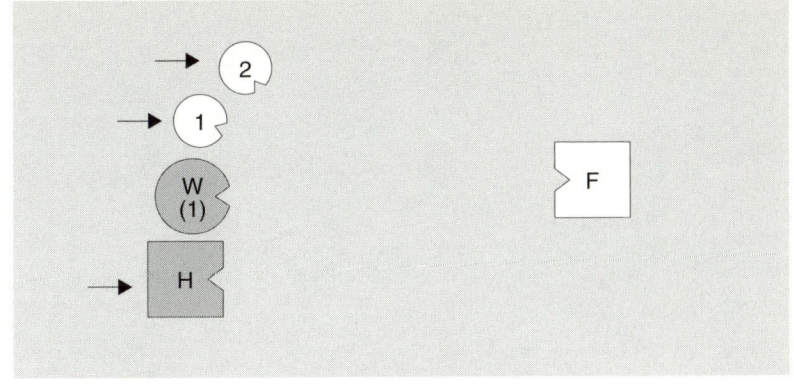

W1   **Wife (First Child of previous constellation)**
H   **Husband**
1   First Child, a daughter
2   Second Child, a daughter

HELLINGER *to the Wife* Say, "Dear Papa."
WIFE Dear Papa.
HELLINGER "This is my husband."
WIFE This is my husband.
HELLINGER "And these are my children."
WIFE And these are my children.
HELLINGER "We have risked it, like you."
WIFE We have risked it, like you.
HELLINGER "Please give us your blessing."
WIFE Please give us your blessing.
HELLINGER *to Father* How is that for you?
FATHER That's good. When my children withdrew, I had a really strong feeling of a tension building. Now that she's said this, that feeling is gone. I feel very calm.
HELLINGER *to Father* Now you retreat a little.

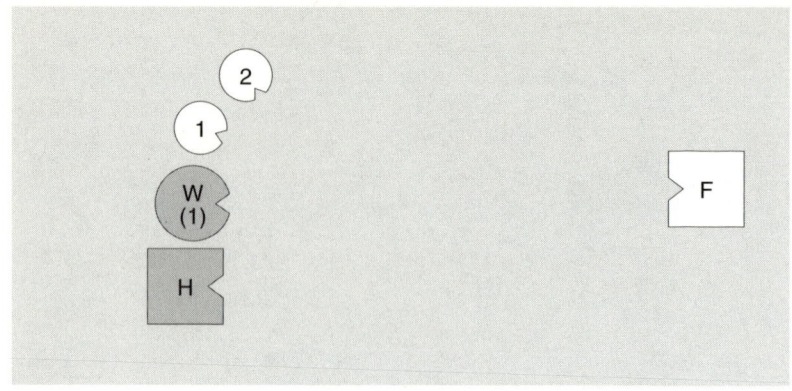

HELLINGER *to husband* Tell her, "I'll hold you as long as I can."

HUSBAND *(very moved)* I'll hold you as long as I can.

HELLINGER Tell your children, too. "I'll hold your mother as long as I can."

HUSBAND I'll hold your mother as long as I can.

HELLINGER "And we'll hold you as long as we can."

HUSBAND And we'll hold you as long as we can.

FIRST CHILD That feels good.

SECOND CHILD That's nice.

WIFE Yes.

HUSBAND That's fine.

HELLINGER *to Wife* Is it all right like that?

WIFE *(nodding)* Yes.

HELLINGER I'll leave it there.

THE RESURRECTION
Grieving for a deceased father

HELLINGER *to Paula, who is grieving for her recently deceased Father* The great Freud observed that when someone dies, those who survive take over something from that person, often something negative. That's a strange thing to do. Do you know how to take care of that?
PAULA Well, first I'd say that you have to live out the negatives and acknowledge them.
HELLINGER You can also let the negative things get buried with your father and resurrect the positives. Agreed?
PAULA Yes.

HELLINGER *to Dorothea* I won't ask you any questions. Just set up a constellation with two representatives, you and death. Okay?
DOROTHEA Yes.
HELLINGER Okay, go ahead. Place them in relationship to each other, according to however it feels. Stay collected within yourself.

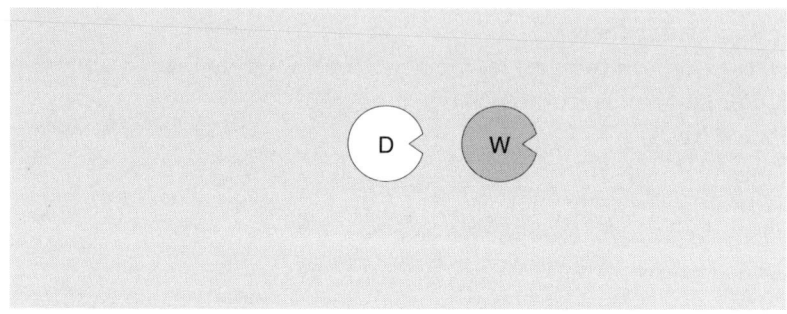

D   Death
W   Woman (Dorothea)

HELLINGER *to the representatives* Stay very collected within yourselves and follow your inner movements.

The two representatives remain where they are for a long time. Hellinger then turns Dorothea's representative to face Death.

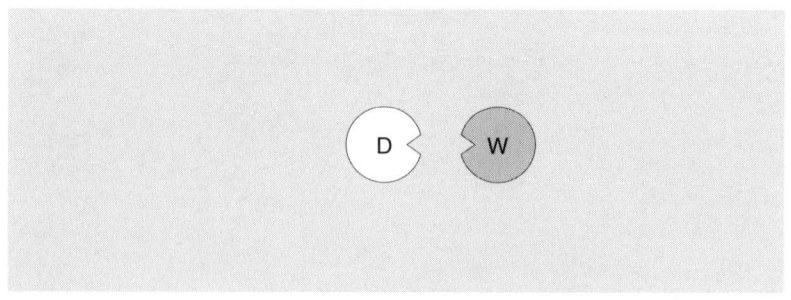

HELLINGER *after a while, to Dorothea's representative* Give in to your movement, whatever it is.

54

Dorothea's representative remains standing motionless. After a while, Hellinger leads her closer to the representative of death.

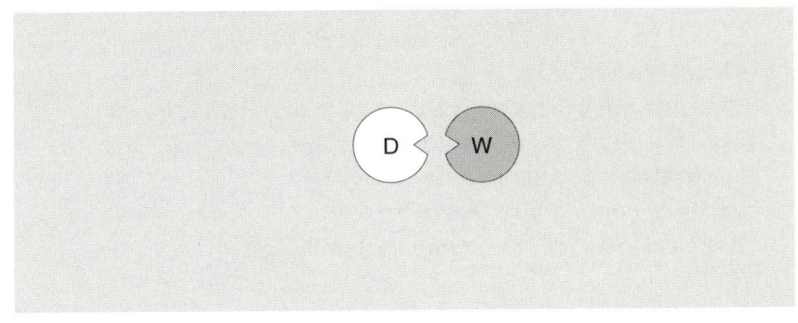

After another pause, Dorothea's representative moves in very close to the death representative. Hellinger bows her head forward so that she is touching Death with her forehead. Death's representative first takes her by the wrists, and then puts her arms around her. Dorothea's representative then puts her arms around Death, and they embrace closely. They remain like that for a long time, and begin to sway together. After a while they release their close embrace, but continue to hold each other's arms.

HELLINGER *to Dorothea's representative* How are you feeling?
WOMAN I was able to get free of the embrace. At first it drew me in, but now I can let it go.
HELLINGER Let go. Follow your impulse.

The two representatives drop their arms, but remain standing close together. Then, Dorothea's representative moves back a step.

HELLINGER *to the Death representative* How is that for you?
DEATH That's okay. I'm here anyway.
HELLINGER *to group* Death stands firm. That's exactly it. Death stands firm.
To Dorothea's representative How are you doing, now?
WOMAN This is also fine.
To Dorothea Is that okay for you?
DOROTHEA Yes, it feels like a release.
HELLINGER Good. That's it, then.
To group I'll tell you a story:

55

The Circle

One who was afflicted asked a companion along the way,
"Could you tell me what really counts for us?"
The other answered:
"The first thing that counts is that we live for a time, which
has a beginning. Before this beginning there has already been
much. When the end comes, it falls back
into the abundance that was before.
As in a closed circle, the beginning and the end
are the same.
So the end of our life joins what was before,
without a break.
As though no time had come between.
We have the time, only now.

The next thing that counts is that the impact we have
during this time withdraws from us as well
as though it belonged to another time
and although we believe we are the doers,
we are, rather, used as a tool
for something beyond us
and then laid aside.
Released, we are complete."

The afflicted one asked
"When we and our works exist for our time
and end,
what counts, when our time comes to a close?"
The other spoke,
"Before and after count as one."

Then the two parted ways and time
and each had pause for thought.

"I TAKE YOU INTO MY HEART"
Non-Hodgkin's lymphomas

HELLINGER *to Gretchen* What's going on with you?
GRETCHEN For the last year I've had highly malignant non-Hodgkin's Lymphomas, and last November I underwent chemotherapy. That's why I'm here. My husband is here, too.
HELLINGER He could come up here and be with you.

Gretchen's husband comes to sit next to her.

HELLINGER *to Gretchen* Have you got any children?
GRETCHEN No, we haven't got any children.
HELLINGER How long have you been married?
GRETCHEN For three years.
HELLINGER Have you got any hope?
GRETCHEN Yes.
HELLINGER No, you haven't got hope.
After a short while What's the effect on you when I say that?
GRETCHEN It's not true!
HELLINGER What shall we do now? We'll set up a constellation of you and the illness. Choose a representative for the illness and place that person. Then, put yourself in relationship to that representative.

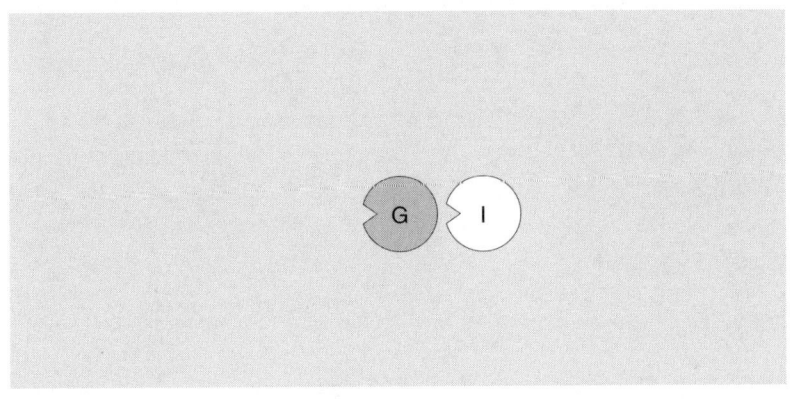

I   Illness
G   **Gretchen**

Both remain motionless for a long time. As Gretchen turns her head towards Hellinger, he tells her to remain collected within herself and to follow her inner sense of movement. After a while, Gretchen reaches behind her and takes her illness by the hand. The representative for the illness moves backwards a bit, but Gretchen holds her tightly with her left hand. As she releases her hand, the illness presses her hands on Gretchen's back. Gretchen then moves first two steps, and then another few steps forwards, turns and looks at the illness.

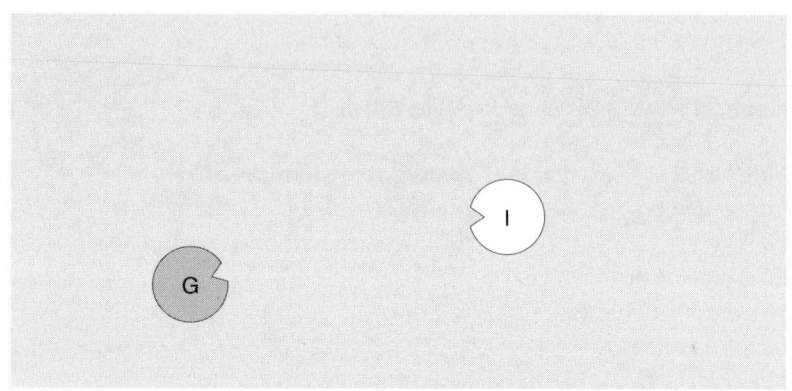

After a while, the illness turns around and moves slowly away.

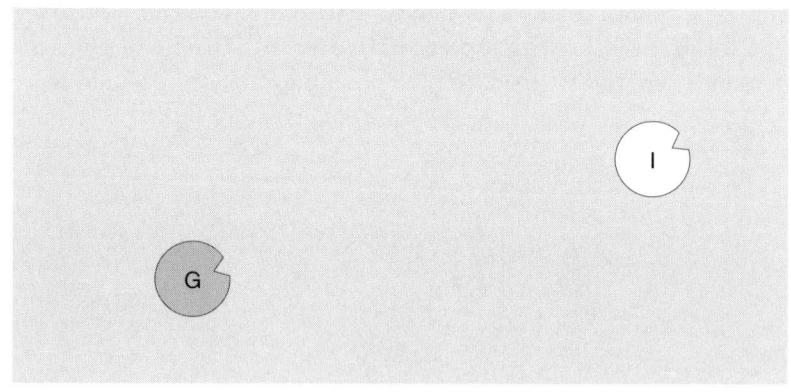

When the illness has moved far away, Gretchen returns to her seat.

HELLINGER Stand up again. If this disease were a person you know, who would it be?
GRETCHEN My mother.

58

HELLINGER Your mother? What happened to her?

GRETCHEN She had two stillbirths before I was born, one in the sixth month, and one baby who died shortly after birth. Up until the time I saw your video about cancer patients, I considered myself the first-born child. When I watched that video, I was aware, for the first time, that I was not the firstborn in our family.

HELLINGER You're talking about others, not about your mother. Collect yourself and see what happens.

Gretchen remains standing motionless for a long time. Then, Hellinger leads her nearer to her mother. She moves up to her and places her hand on her mother's shoulder from behind. The mother turns to her and they embrace warmly, with a slight rocking motion. After a while they release each other from the embrace and look at one another. Then, the mother moves a couple of steps backwards.

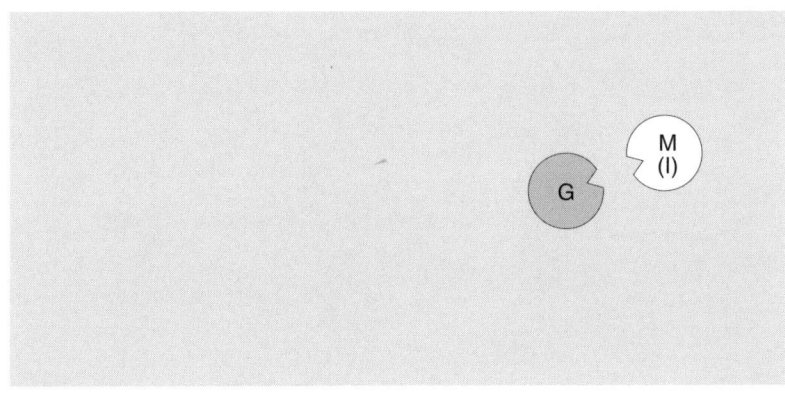

M   Mother

HELLINGER Okay, that was it.

Gretchen sits down next to Hellinger. Her husband puts his arm around her and Hellinger holds her hand.

HELLINGER *after a while, to Gretchen* Close your eyes and say, "I take you into my heart."

GRETCHEN I take you into my heart.

HELLINGER *after a pause* Is it good like that?

GRETCHEN It's blissful.

HELLINGER I'll tell you something about illness. They are sometimes messengers of love. If you allow them to come, they may be friendly. Okay?

GRETCHEN Yes.

HELLINGER Good. That's all.

SONJA I'm here because I have had four accidents which have had major effects on my life.

HELLINGER What happened?

SONJA When I was six months old, I fell down a flight of stairs with my grandmother – there are always stairs involved – and from that accident I have a cyst in my head. That one doesn't affect me. At seven, I fell down by myself the first time. That time I was paralyzed for an hour, completely paralyzed, and I couldn't speak a word. After an hour that passed.

The next accident happened when I was 27. *She falters and can barely speak. She begins to cry.* I had encephalitis, but went to work anyway. At work I fell down a flight of stairs. When I woke up I was in the hospital and had a severe epileptic fit. In the hospital they said that I didn't have epilepsy, and that I wouldn't ever have an attack like that again. They said it was ridiculous, and there was no epilepsy involved. After a month, I was released from the hospital as fully recovered. Two months later it started again. There was a man and he introduced me to his father as the woman he loved and wanted to marry. That night the attacks started up again. Shortly thereafter I was pregnant. I was pregnant three times, and I aborted all three times. I always have the attacks in the night. I went on like that for years. Eleven years ago, my father died, and since then I haven't been able to leave the house.

Sonja's story is related very dramatically and with difficulty.

HELLINGER Look at me.

SONJA Yes.

HELLINGER Something doesn't add up.

SONJA I know something's not right, but I don't know what.

HELLINGER Something is definitely not right.

SONJA What isn't right?

HELLINGER That I don't know. But someone who behaves as you did just now, is avoiding a guilt of some kind. That's a non-acceptance of guilt.

SONJA I'm guilty?

HELLINGER A person who behaves in this way, as you do, is usually repressing a guilt, is not accepting a guilt. Now, how is that?

SONJA I don't know what I should say. I don't know what it is. There's a lie somewhere, but I don't know what it is.

HELLINGER Exactly. There's a total lie there. That's exactly it.

SONJA Yes, but I don't know what. I don't know if the lie comes from me, or if I've believed a lie that someone else told me. I just don't know.

HELLINGER The image I have is that it comes from you.

SONJA It comes from me?

HELLINGER Yes.

SONJA Then, the epilepsy is a lie?

HELLINGER Sometimes, a disease is easier to bear than the truth.

SONJA I've thought of that. I've thought that I create these attacks so that I'm completely unconscious. Then I can't be aware of anything.

HELLINGER That kind of insinuation leads away. Where is the guilt? For example, who have you wronged, and in what way?

SONJA I didn't respect my mother. I think I wanted to take my father away from her. I wanted my father all for myself.

HELLINGER No, that's not sufficient for something like this.

SONJA When I was a child, a couple of times I took a knife and stood behind the door praying to God that my mother would die.

HELLINGER That's it then. Now it's coming out. Let's set up a constellation of you and your mother.

Sonja chooses a representative for her mother and places her facing herself at some distance. Then she takes a few more steps backwards.

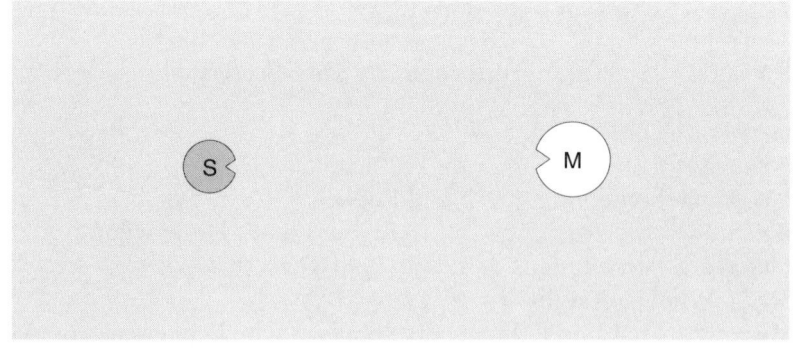

M   Mother
S   **Sonja**

HELLINGER *to Sonja* Remain very calm. Open your mouth slightly and breathe normally. Look at her calmly.

After a while Sonja moves another step backwards.

HELLINGER How's the mother feeling?
MOTHER I'm starting to slip away inside. At first I liked my daughter a lot. I was really there for her. I couldn't figure out what was going on with her.

Hellinger chooses a representative for Sonja's father, and places him to the right of the mother.

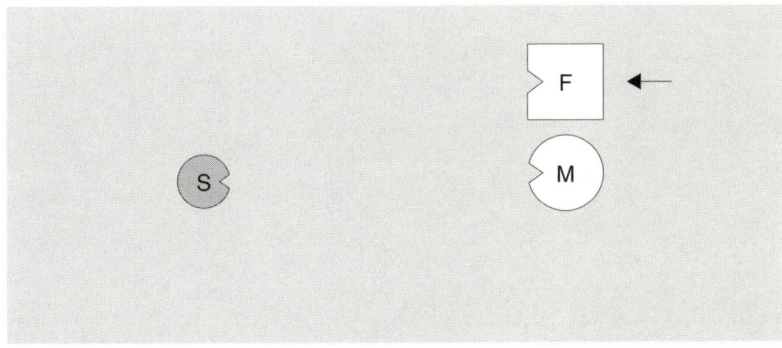

F   Father

As soon as the man is standing next to her, the mother becomes very agitated and pulls away from him.

MOTHER That's not okay.
HELLINGER *to Father* What's going on with you?
FATHER I'm not feeling anything special.
MOTHER I feel like praying to God to make him disappear.
HELLINGER Aha.

Hellinger turns the father and mother so that they are looking at one another. The woman backs away from her husband.

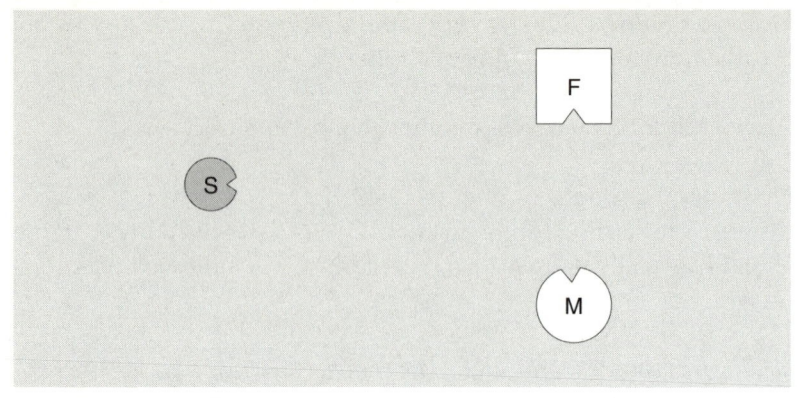

HELLINGER *to Sonja* Turn around.

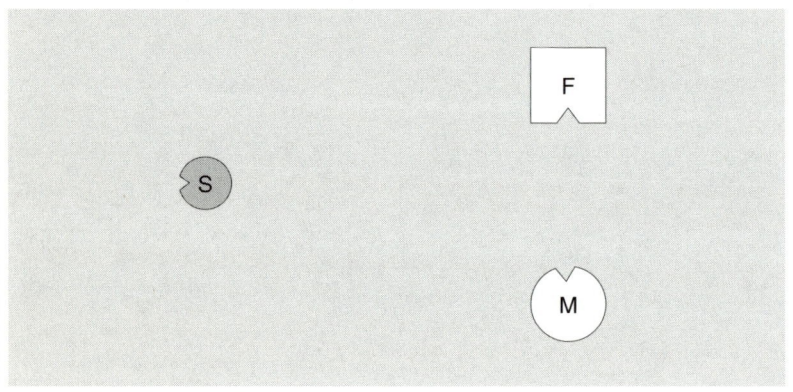

HELLINGER *to Mother* What's going on with you?

MOTHER I'm breaking out in a sweat, and I'm shaking. I'm incredibly afraid.

HELLINGER *to Father* And you?

FATHER I still don't feel anything in particular. I don't know what's going on with her.

HELLINGER *to group* Judging by the reactions here, I would suspect a double shift. The mother has feelings which belong to another person, and that are directed towards someone else. The mother has taken over these feelings and directs her reaction towards her husband. He's completely helpless in that situation. There is an entanglement here.

To Mother Does that make sense to you?

64

MOTHER Yes.

HELLINGER *to Sonja* How are you feeling now?

SONJA With my back turned to them I feel very calm.

HELLINGER Okay, now turn around again.

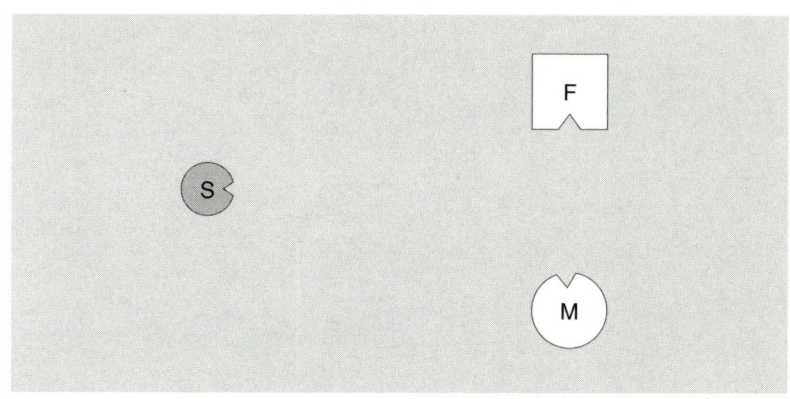

HELLINGER Tell your mother, "I'll leave this with you."

SONJA I'll leave this with you.

HELLINGER "I'm only the little one."

SONJA I'm only the little one.

HELLINGER Tell your father the same thing.

SONJA I'll leave this with you. I'm only the little one.

HELLINGER Turn around again.

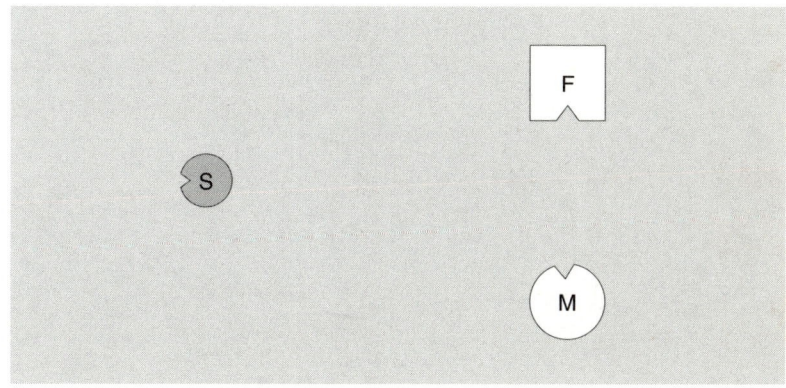

HELLINGER How is that now?

SONJA I'd like to just hop away. So jolly.

HELLINGER That's right.

Sonja laughs.

HELLINGER You can do that now. Okay, that's it.

"WITH YOU, IT TASTES GOOD"
Eating disorder

HELLINGER Why are you here?

MARION I'm not so ill. I'm bulimic (an eating disorder characterized by vomiting) and I have anxiety attacks. I've been bulimic for seven years, and the anxiety attacks have always been there.

HELLINGER Were you ever anorexic?

MARION Not really.

HELLINGER Are you married?

MARION Yes. My husband is here, too.

HELLINGER He could come and sit by you. You get a more complete picture of a person when their spouse is sitting next to them. Have you got any children?

MARION No.

HELLINGER What happened in your family of origin?

MARION I'm an illegitimate child. My father took off after I was born. I don't know him. My mother got married when I was six years old. I grew up thinking that this man was my real father. Up to the time when my mother married my stepfather, I had been living with my grandparents. My grandfather was a very important person in my life. He died when I was 17. I also have a brother. He's the son of my mother and my stepfather.

HELLINGER We'll just set up one person. Who do we need to set up?

MARION My father?

HELLINGER Of course. Choose someone to represent your father. *When she has chosen and placed the representative* Now place yourself in relation to him.

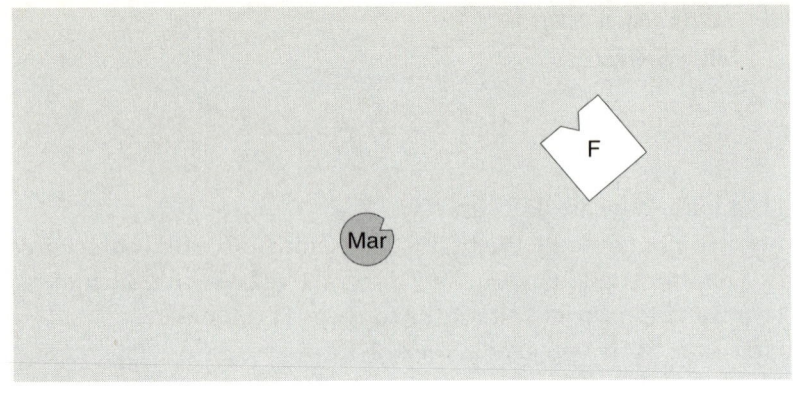

F   Father
M   **Marion**

HELLINGER *to father's representative* Follow your own impulse, also in where to look. Remain collected within yourself and give in to any impulses you feel.

The father's representative takes one sideways step towards his daughter. Hesitating, he takes one more step and then a third. Then he remains standing. He doesn't risk a look at his daughter.

HELLINGER *to Marion* Say to him, "Please, Daddy."
MARION Please, Daddy.
HELLINGER "Please."
MARION *(very emotionally)* Please.

The father's representative moves sideways a bit closer to her. The he turns to her and puts his left arm around her. Marion weeps and looks down at the floor. Then, she raises her eyes to him.

HELLINGER *to Marion* Look at him.

She turns somewhat and her father drops his arm. Marion moves one step backwards and the two stand facing each other.

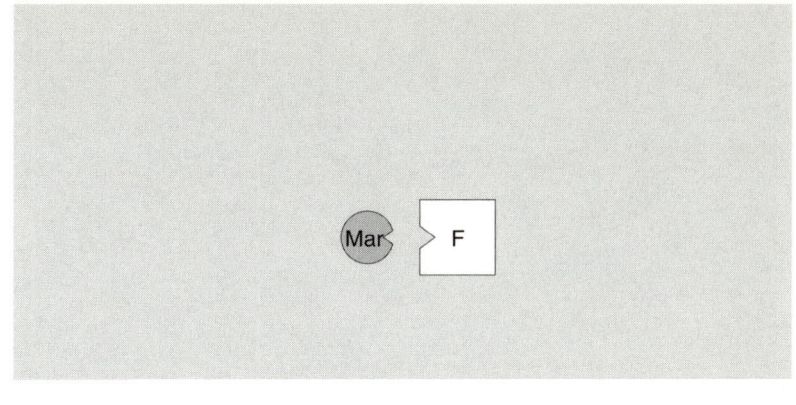

HELLINGER *to Marion* Say, "Please, Daddy."
MARION *sobbing* Please, Daddy, come to me.

The father's representative takes a step closer. Marion throws her arms around his neck and embraces him warmly.

HELLINGER *after a while, to Marion* Breathe deeply.
MARION *(weeping)* He's not here by me, I can feel it. He isn't taking me.

She releases her embrace. The father steps back away.

HELLINGER *to Father* You have to say something to her.
FATHER I'm here by you now.
HELLINGER *to group* Here you can see the pain of an interrupted movement. The father has to meet her halfway. There's no other way, because she can't do it.
To Father Tell her, "I'm sorry, and now I take you as my daughter."
FATHER I'm sorry and now I take you as my daughter.
HELLINGER You'll have to take her. Nothing else will help here. The father has to make the move towards her.

The father's representative moves towards Marion and they embrace warmly. As this is going on, Hellinger chooses a representative for Marion's mother and places her where Marion can see her.

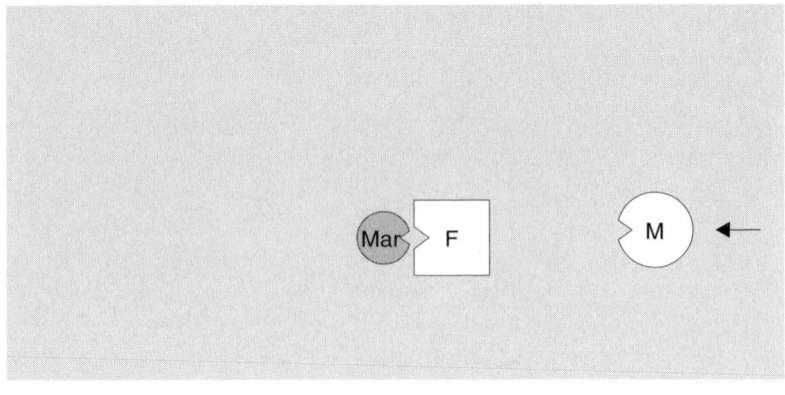

M   Mother

HELLINGER *to Marion* Tell her, "Mama, I take him now as my father."
You can keep holding on to him while you say that. Look at her and
say, "Mama, I take him now as my father."
MARION *(emotionally)* Mama, this is my father. Now I take him.

*She cries and laughs at the same time and remains embracing her father.
The mother laughs as well.*

HELLINGER Say it once more, loudly!
MARION I'm proud of him, too.

*After a while, Hellinger leads the mother to stand next to the father. She
puts her arm around him and then the three all embrace.*

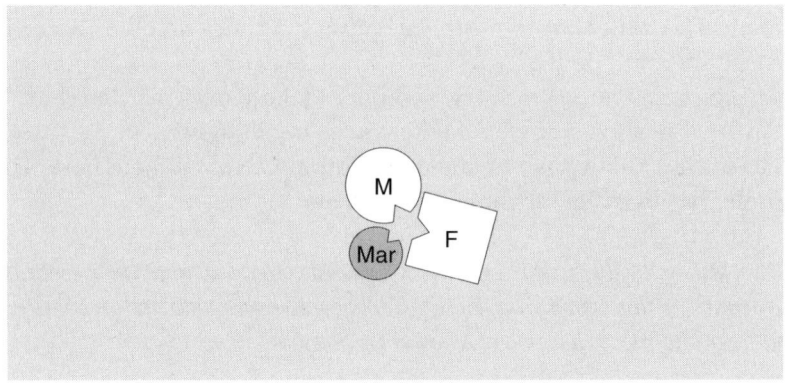

HELLINGER *after a while to Marion* Now tell your mother, "I take you and I take him."

MARION I take you and I take him.

HELLINGER *to group as the three embrace* I'll explain one of the secrets of bulimia. It's been demonstrated wonderfully here. A person who is bulimic is only allowed to take from the mother. It's forbidden to take anything from the father. Therefore, she eats but vomits it up again. In telling her mother, I take you and I take him, she can retain her food.

HELLINGER *to Marion* Tell her once more, "I take you and I take him."

MARION I take you and I take him.

HELLINGER "I keep you in and I keep him in."

As she hesitates Say it once, just to try it out.

MARION I keep you in and I keep him in.

HELLINGER "With you it tastes good and with him it tastes good."

MARION *laughing* With you it tastes good and with him it tastes good.

HELLINGER That was it. That's the healing of bulimia. It's always the same.

Laughter in the group.

HELLINGER *to Marion as she sits next to him again* The next time you have a bulimic attack, this is what to do: Spread all the food you want to eat out on the table. Then play a little game with your husband. He takes a teaspoon and you tell him what you want to eat first. He takes a spoonful and feeds you. As he feeds you, you say, "Daddy, with you it tastes good." Then, you eat as much as you want. Take as much as you want. That would be a nice exercise that will also bring you and your husband close.

Marion and her husband look at each other and laugh.

HELLINGER Okay, that's it.

PARTICIPANT You asked her if she was anorexic. How would the solution for anorexia be different?

HELLINGER Bulimia often follows anorexia. Sometimes the bulimia appears alone, as with her, and sometimes it's a consequence of anorexia. In that case it would have a different meaning. In that case, eating says "I'm alive", and vomiting says, "I'm disappearing". The resolution would be for such a bulimic person to say, while eating, "I'm staying!"

A Picture
Fatal accident involving husband and child

Hellinger What's your issue?

Erika Two years ago my husband and child were killed in an accident. I'm here to try to learn how to live with that.

Hellinger How many children have you got?

Erika The one child. Earlier I had a miscarriage.

Hellinger So your husband and child both died in the accident. What happened?

Erika It was a car accident with a train. My husband didn't see a train that was coming on a side track – a track where normally there were no trains. It was just 300 meters from where we lived.

Hellinger We'll do a constellation of you, your husband, and your child.

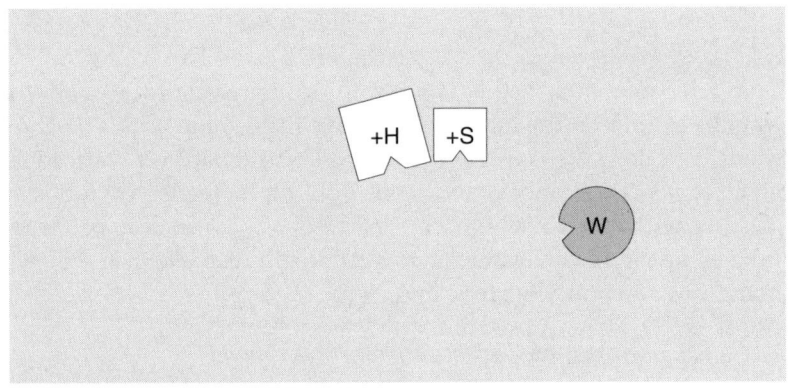

+H   Husband, killed in accident
W   Wife (Erika)
+S   Son, killed with his father in accident

Hellinger *to wife's representative* How are you feeling?

Wife I'm cold. I feel drawn forward. I feel pulled over there.

Hellinger How about the husband?

Husband I feel warm towards my son. I feel pulled forward, but something is holding my feet. I feel very heavy.

Hellinger And the son?

72

CHILD My legs are shaking. My right side is very warm, but somehow it's too close for me. My left foot is weak, and the right feels as if it wants to push off.

HELLINGER *to wife's representative* Follow your impulse.

She moves several steps forward and turns around.

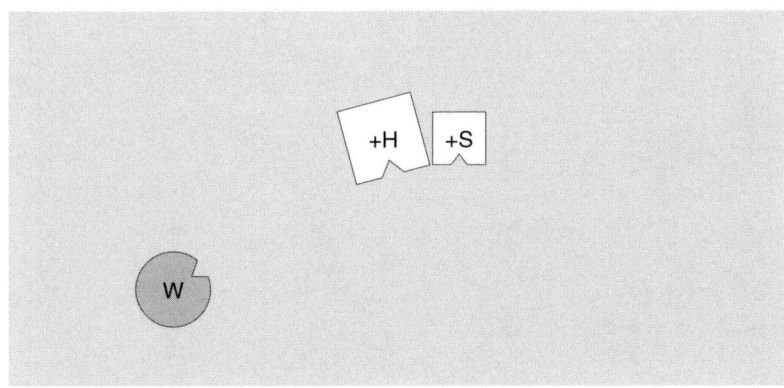

HELLINGER How do you feel now?

WIFE Better. I can breathe easier.

HELLINGER And the husband?

HUSBAND Not much has changed for me. Perhaps that pulling forwards is gone, but not much has changed.

HELLINGER *to son* What about you?

CHILD Things have got a bit easier. I feel like turning.

HELLINGER Go ahead. Do whatever you want.

He moves several steps away from his father and turns towards his mother.

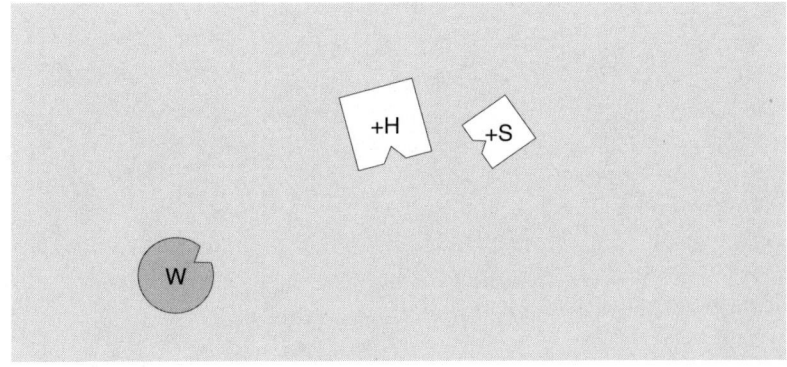

HELLINGER Like that?
CHILD Yes, that's about right.
HELLINGER And for the father?
HUSBAND I feel like I have to go after him.
HELLINGER Do it.

He moves and stands next to the son.

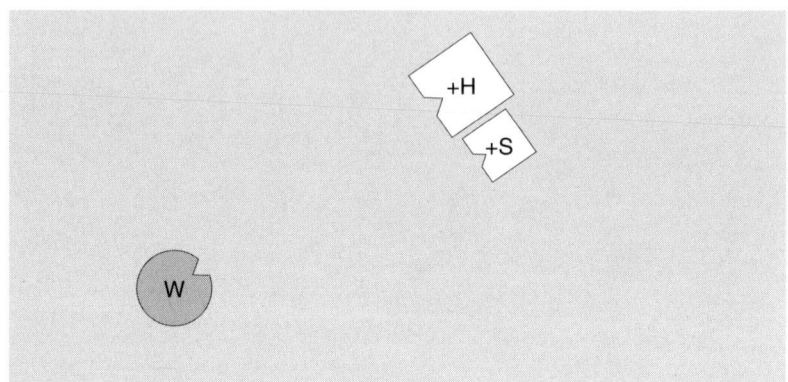

HELLINGER *to son* How is that now?
CHILD That's too close for me. The direction towards my mother fits, but my father is too close, and somehow I'm not connected to him.

Hellinger leads the husband in the direction where he originally felt drawn.

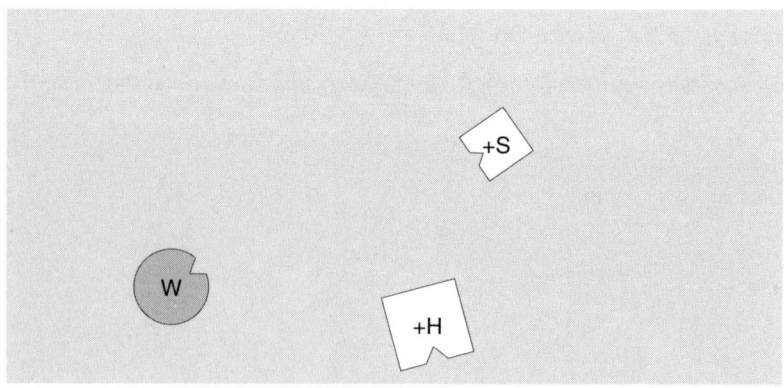

HELLINGER *to husband* How is that?

HUSBAND Good. I feel free. The heaviness is gone from my feet and I can stand normally.

HELLINGER *to son* And for you?

CHILD I feel a lot lighter and I'm being pulled towards my mother.

Hellinger leads him to his mother and places him near her on the left side.

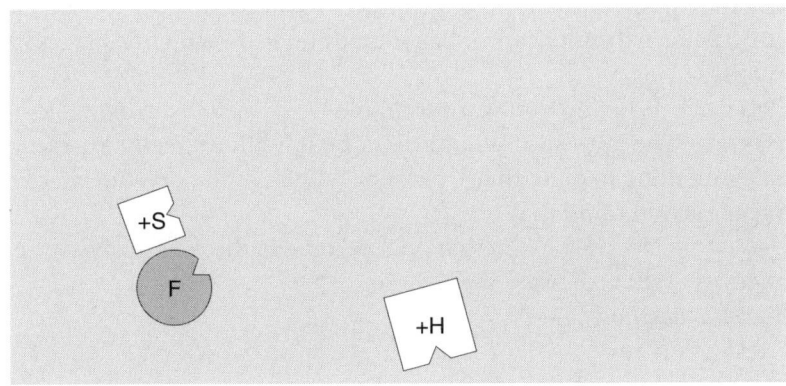

HELLINGER *to Mother* Put your arm around him.

To son How is that?

CHILD Pleasant.

HELLINGER And for the mother?

WIFE That feels right.

HELLINGER *to Erika* I'll leave it there. Have you got that picture?

ERIKA Yes.

HELLINGER What is your issue?

MARTINA Three years ago I was in this clinic as a cancer patient and had the opportunity to hear a lecture by Mr. Kurz. This lecture led me to believe that my cancer has something to do with my soul, with my life.

HELLINGER What do you want from me?

MARTINA The issue, as I would describe it, without really knowing, has something to do with my parents, with my mother, who rejected me. *(Crying)* I think that …

HELLINGER No, no, no. Let that go. Look me in the eyes. Can you see my eyes? What color are they?

MARTINA *laughing* Grey.

HELLINGER Grey?

MARTINA *laughing loudly* Yes.

HELLINGER *to group* I just played a little trick, that shows you how to get someone out of that kind of emotional feeling. When a person pulls back and closes their eyes and dives into an emotion, as she just did here, that feeling has no value. There's no strength in that and the feelings that count are those with strength.

To Martina I wonder if you really need anything at all. You're healthy.

MARTINA Yes, but I don't know if there's not still something there that could get me.

HELLINGER Your zeal does you the most harm. *Laughter in the group.*
To group Yes, her zeal is harmful to her.
To Martina That's egocentric. "I want …" The soul works differently. *After a short pause* I'll give you one tip. It's the entire therapy. Say "Dear Mommy."

Martina shakes her head.

HELLINGER Exactly. It'll take a year before you're able to do that, but it's the best exercise. Okay?

MARTINA Yes.

HELLINGER *to group* I'd like to say something about cancer. Cancer in women is often connected to an unwillingness to take and honor their mothers. Many cancer patients would rather die than bow down before their mother. The complaint that the mother rejected them or whatever is just a way to justify this refusal. It has nothing to do with the real mother. I'm not too interested in that.

To Martina Okay?

Martina nods.

THE SUBSTITUTE
Anxiety and panic attacks, depression, cancer, and a suicidal daughter

HELLINGER What is it?

LUCIA I have anxiety attacks, panic attacks, depression, and cancer. My daughter has made a few suicide attempts. My mother's first husband had to shoot himself because he was a Nazi.

HELLINGER Who forced him to do that?

LUCIA The political situation. It was his choice of death. He was to be shot but he could shoot himself if he wanted.

HELLINGER What had he done?

LUCIA I don't know that.

HELLINGER What happened to your mother?

LUCIA She was married to that man and had a son. She brought this son with her into our family, I mean with my father. He was not respected, and was pushed off to the side. My mother allowed herself to be humiliated and beaten by my father.

HELLINGER We'll set up a constellation with two people your mother and her first husband. Set them up according to your inner feeling right now.

M   Mother
+M1H   Mother's first husband, was forced to shoot himself.

HELLINGER *as he sees that Lucia is having difficulty setting up the constellation* I will set up the representatives for you.

78

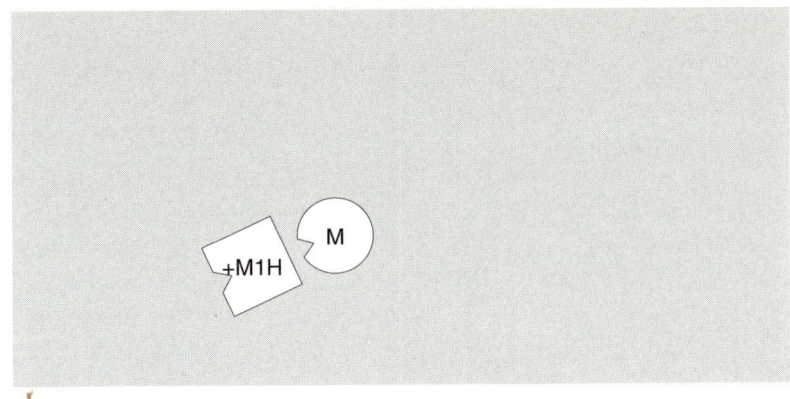

HELLINGER *to the mother's representative* How is that for you?
MOTHER It's weird looking at this back in front of me.
HELLINGER How do you feel?
MOTHER I can't see his face. I can't see the person.
HELLINGER *to first husband* How are you doing?
MOTHER'S FIRST HUSBAND Before, it was very threatening. Now I can breathe, and I feel pretty indifferent.

Hellinger chooses a representative for Lucia and places her behind her mother.

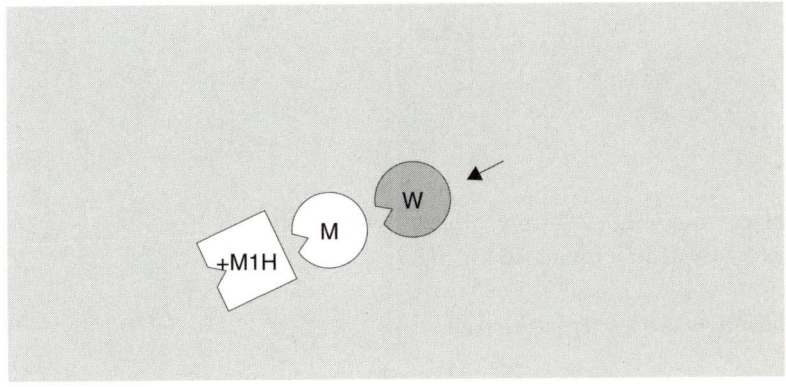

W   Woman (Lucia)

HELLINGER *to Lucia's representative* How is that?
WOMAN Bah! All walled in. (*Sighing*) I can't move forward.
HELLINGER I'll take the mother out.

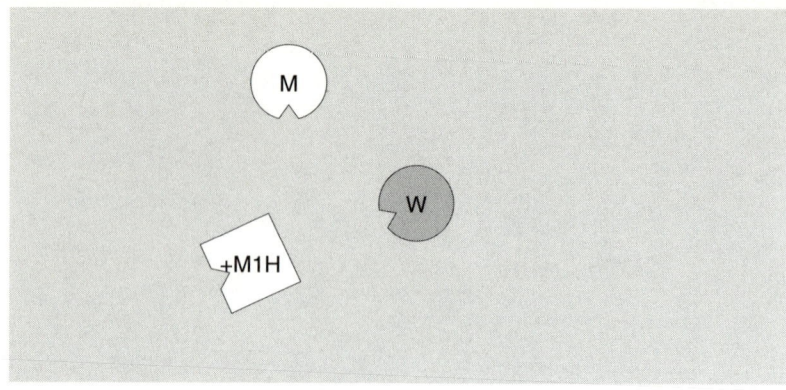

HELLINGER *to Lucia's representative* How is that?
WOMAN There's more air and more room to move.

Hellinger leads her forward behind her mother's first husband.

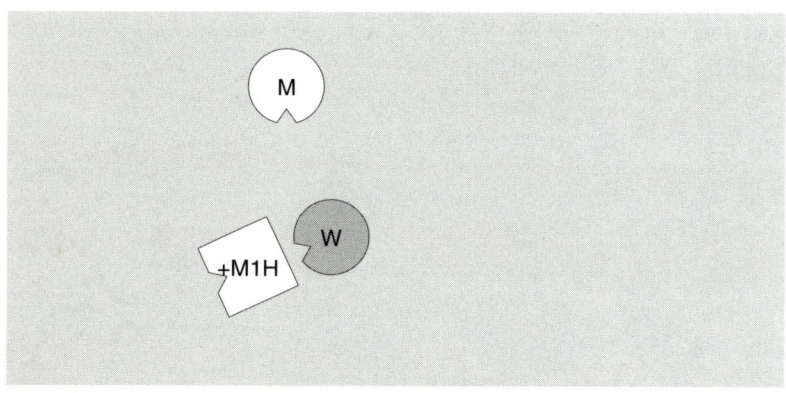

HELLINGER *to Lucia's representative* How is that?
WOMAN That's too close for me.

Hellinger moves her back a step.

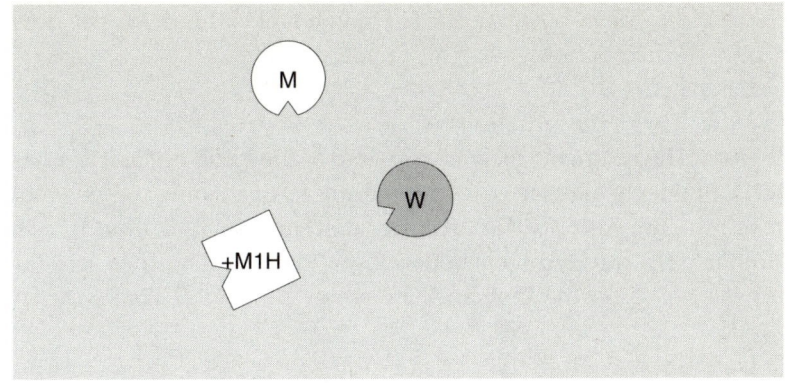

WOMAN That's better.

HELLINGER *to Mother* How are you feeling, now that your daughter is standing here, better or worse?

MOTHER I feel better I can see my daughter.

HELLINGER *to Lucia* Do you understand this picture?

LUCIA I don't really understand it, because he's not my father. He's my brother's father. I don't understand why I'm following him.

HELLINGER So that your mother will stay.

LUCIA *after a while* I still don't understand why I have the feeling that I'm trying to disappear through my illness, and my daughter through her suicide attempts.

Hellinger chooses a representative for Lucia's daughter and places her behind her grandmother's first husband. He moves Lucia's representative over next to her mother.

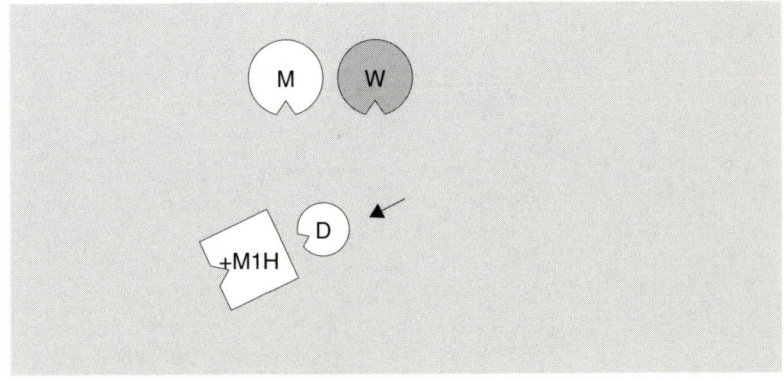

D   Daughter, who has attempted suicide several times.

HELLINGER *to Lucia's representative* Do you feel better or worse, now?

WOMAN Much better.

HELLINGER Exactly.

To Lucia That's the situation.

To group The mother clearly bears some of the guilt, not just her husband. She feels like she owes something to this death, or she wants to follow him into death. Then, her daughter says, "I'll do it." The mother pulls out and feels better. Now the next daughter sees that her mother is on the line, and she says, "I'll do it." That's the dynamic.

To Lucia I'll leave it there.

To the representatives That was it, thank you.

HELLINGER *after a while, to group* What I've done here was risky of course.

To Lucia How are you feeling?

LUCIA I'm horrified that my daughter is perhaps trying to take over something from me. How can I resolve that?

HELLINGER I'll wait a while. We'll let that have its effect first. Then, later, you can come back. But first, you have to let it work in your soul. And ask, sometime, how involved your mother was.

LUCIA My daughter was also abused by her father.

HELLINGER That's another issue, and it diverts the energy here. Okay, that's all.

There are basically two dynamics in families that lead to life-threatening illness or to serious accidents indicating that a person is trying to disappear, to leave.

The first dynamic is "I'll follow you into death." That was my image when Lucia said that her mother's first husband was forced to shoot himself. His wife couldn't remain unaffected by that. Most probably she said, "I'll follow you into death." That is even more likely if she was also guilty. That would be the soul's movement then, and it would be appropriate. When something like that has happened, you cannot step in to change that movement. If there was criminal guilt on the mother's part, it would probably have been appropriate for her to die too, or to kill herself. Otherwise, of course, it's not appropriate. If it's just the woman following the man she loved, then her death isn't appropriate.

When a child becomes aware that his or her mother is drawn to leave, the child steps into the mother's place. In this constellation, the mother didn't have any feelings. She was not facing up to something, perhaps her own guilt. She pushed that off on to her husband. Then, the child comes along and says, "I'll do it for you." The child then has a child of her own who also says, "I'll do it in your place, Mama." This is the other dynamic that leads to suicide or critical illness. It says, "Better me than you. It's better for me to die than you. I'll disappear instead of you."

The fantasy that lies behind this is that the child believes that the destructive action will rescue the loved one. As this sequence shows, however, it just gets pushed from generation to generation and nothing is resolved. No one is rescued. It is only pushed on, and always on to the weakest one. It is pushed into the next generation when someone refuses to accept their fate or their guilt.

In taking this over, the child also has a feeling of power, and feels like the savior in the family. The child is inflated, but it stems from love. Because the child is acting out of love, he or she feels no sense of guilt, it is all done with a clear conscience. But behind this conscience, which we feel through love, there is an archaic conscience we cannot feel, because it lies too deep. We can only recognize this conscience by its effects. When a child, out of love, attempts a rescue action, this deep conscience in the background dooms the child to failure because the child is presuming to do something inappropriate for his or her position as a child. It is not the task of a child to rescue a parent in this way. The child would be acting as if he or she were the big one and the parent is like a child. That is an offense to the natural order of things.

No
Cancer

HELLINGER What's the issue?
MARGARET I've been suffering for many years from depression and anxiety states. Eight months ago I got cancer.
HELLINGER Close your eyes and open your mouth. Let your head bow down slightly. Let your head loose. Breathe in and out deeply. *After a while* Say to yourself, inside, "Yes."

After an inner struggle, she shakes her head, no.

HELLINGER *to group* That's one of the causes of cancer. Could you see it? It's easier to die.
To Margaret Okay, I've showed you. There's nothing else I can do.
To group What I have done here is a strange form of the work that takes place silently, in secret, without anything being exposed. You can get indications from the body language and you just give the soul a nudge. It brings something into consciousness or just brings something up. Now the soul has a new strength and a new orientation, as well as a freedom that wasn't there before. Now the soul can decide what to do and the therapist stays out of the way. The therapist isn't allowed to tamper with this, so he pulls back.
To someone who is holding and comforting Margaret It would be better for you to leave her alone. That comforting is weakening her.
To Margaret Can you feel that?
MARGARET I feel very strong.
HELLINGER *to group* She doesn't need comforting. What happened earlier, is what brings her strength. Nobody can replace that or strengthen it, that's not possible.

I would like to say something about the attitude of the therapist in this work. I don't have to give that too much thought, because I rely on an old friend of mine, Laotse, who is long since dead. He spoke of the effects of retreating into the empty center.

One who retreats into the empty center has no intentions and no fear. Without taking any action, things begin to come into order of their own accord. This is an appropriate attitude for a therapist – to retreat into the empty center. You don't need to close your eyes to do this. The empty center is connected, not closed off. You retreat without fear, and that is really important. Anybody who is worried about what might happen can pack it in right there. And, you have to remain without intent, even without any intent to heal.

Within the empty center, which is, of course, only an image, you are connected. Within these connections, if you allow it, images suddenly appear – images of resolution. These are the images you follow. You can also make mistakes, that is clear, but the mistakes take care of themselves through an echo that comes. So, the therapist needn't be perfect in this work, and does not presume to be superior in any way. You only have to be still and quiet in this center, and the work can succeed.

It is humility that is important here. The absence of a goal agrees to an ill person as he or she is, agrees to the illness as it is, and agrees to fate as it is. No one is stronger of more able to handle a fate than the person whose fate it is. A therapist is only someone who is there and who provides a space in which the patient can develop strength. What has an effect, however, is non-intervention and being there.

Presumption
Diabetes, a brother's suicide

HELLINGER *to Helen* What is it?

HELEN I've had diabetes for 23 years. The disease is very difficult to regulate as it swings from very high to very low. Sometimes it disappears for a week or two and then is very bad again for a while.

HELLINGER Did something happen 23 years ago?

HELEN My brother died.

HELLINGER How?

HELEN He killed himself. *(Crying)* I can't forget it. It's always there.

HELLINGER Are you angry with him?

HELEN No.

HELLINGER You are angry with him.

HELEN I've never felt like I was angry with him.

HELLINGER He didn't accept help from you. Sometimes people feel that as an insult.

HELEN No, I didn't even know how bad things were for him. For a long time things went along with him just on the edge.

HELLINGER Set up a constellation with two people, you and your brother.

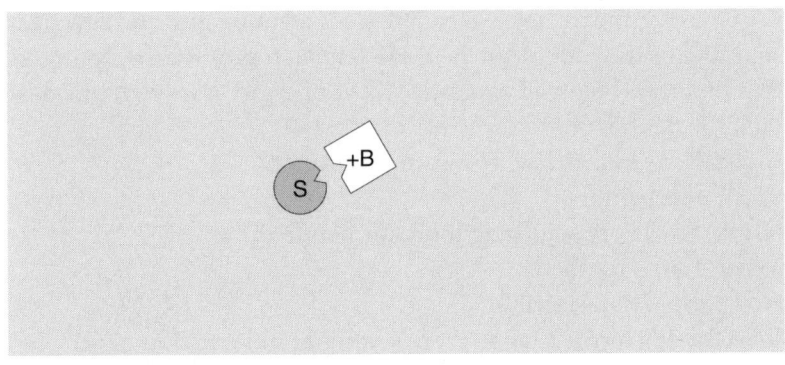

S   **Sister (Helen)**   +B   Brother, committed suicide

The two look at each other for a long time.

HELLINGER *to deceased Brother* Pull back, just according to your own sense, and turn around.

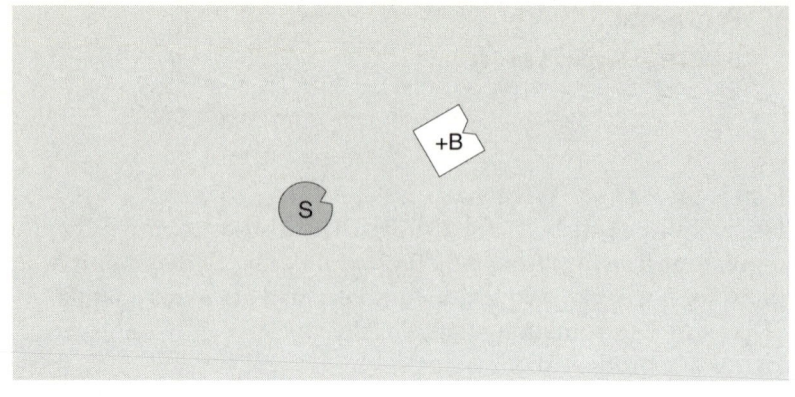

HELLINGER *to deceased Brother* How is that?

BROTHER A lot better than before. That was much too close.

HELLINGER Exactly.

BROTHER I could hardly breathe.

HELLINGER She's being presumptuous.

To Helen There's a fairy tale from the Brothers Grimm collection that has to do with a doctor who makes a pact with death. Whenever this doctor was called to a sickbed, he could see immediately whether the patient would live or die. If death was standing at the head of the bed, the patient would live. If death was standing at the foot of the bed, the doctor knew that the patient would die.

One day, the doctor was called to see a young girl, and saw death standing at the foot of the bed. He felt such pity for the young girl that he turned the bed around. The young girl survived, but death took the doctor.

To Helen's representative How are you doing?

SISTER I feel empty.

HELLINGER There's nothing more for you to do.

SISTER That's it exactly.

HELLINGER That's terrible.

To Helen It's terrible when there's nothing more to do.

Hellinger turns Helen's representative around.

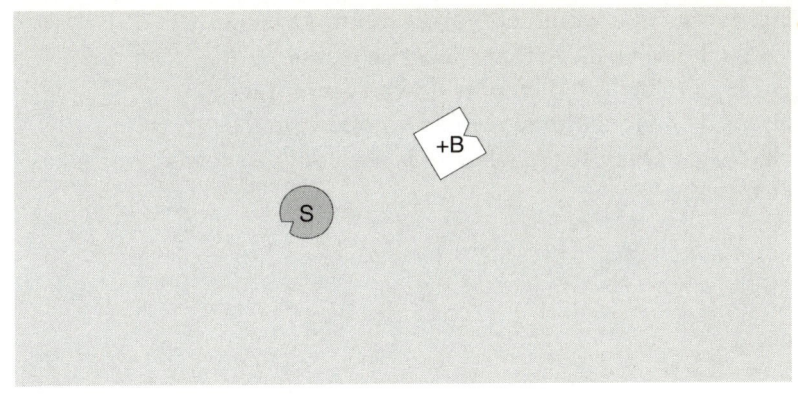

HELLINGER *to Helen's representative* How is that for you?

SISTER Very good.

HELLINGER *to Helen* What do you have to say to that?

HELEN I don't know what to do with that.

HELLINGER That's right. Nobody gives up such a lofty position so easily, judging over life and death.

HELEN I don't think that I was trying to judge.

HELLINGER That's what came out. You presumed to stand in his way.

HELEN I don't think so.

HELLINGER That's how you set it up.

HELEN I was only standing close to him, nothing more.

HELLINGER That's how it is with standing close. I'll stick to that picture.

HELLINGER *to group* What would have happened if her brother had stayed alive to please her. How would his life have been?

To a participant How would his life have been?

PARTICIPANT Probably worse.

HELLINGER Worse. Worse than now.

HELEN I can't believe that.

HELLINGER Okay, that's how it is. It's easier to have diabetes than to give up your belief.

HELEN I don't want the diabetes either.

HELLINGER I'll give you a different image. Imagine that you're lying beside your brother in his grave.

HELEN I don't want to do that, either.

HELLINGER That would be a great comfort to him.
HELEN I don't believe that's what he wants.
HELLINGER Really? Then why do you act as if it is?
HELEN For a long time I wanted to follow him.
HELLINGER Okay, that's where it is. I think I've showed you. Okay?
HELEN Yes.

I would like to say something about suicide.

The first thing is that it is unavoidable in some cases, it is the only thing that can happen, and we have to respect that. Our interference stems from a belief that life is the most precious thing and that we have to keep people alive. As a rule, people commit suicide out of love, but it is rarely honored in the family as an act of love.

In my book, "The Orders of Love", I described one situation where this is made very clear. There was an old pediatrician in one of my courses. He was 70 years old but was still grieving for his son who had hanged himself at age 12. He had sent his son to do some shopping, and when the boy came home, he had dropped the bag and spilled everything out on the steps. His father had swatted him in punishment, and the son hanged himself that night.

A year later the doctor came to another course. We went for a walk together and talked about this. I told him that his son's suicide may have had to do with love. At that moment he suddenly remembered that a few days before this event, his wife had announced her pregnancy. This son's reaction was a loud, "But there's not enough room!" His suicide was making space for the new child.

The doctor also told me later that during that night, as he was lying in bed with his wife, he had suddenly had an eerie feeling of lightness. That is the way things happen sometimes.

At the end of the course he said, "Now I'm sitting on a calm lake." He was at peace with his son, in love.

PARTICIPANT Are suicides and suicide attempts the same thing, or do you see them as different?

HELLINGER No, a suicide attempt is headed in the same direction. There are cases, however, when a suicide is prevented, that the person is very relieved afterwards. Sometimes the suicide attempt seems to be a demonstration of love that then frees the person from their burden. That sometimes seems to release the person from this fate. Sometimes, but not always.

To group I'm not saying that you shouldn't try to prevent a suicide. But there are situations where you can't prevent it. For example, if a suicidal person is attempting to atone for a serious crime, there's a different dynamic. It's more like an offering to the victim, like bowing down before the victim. You can see it from this perspective. If a person has killed another, or committed a very serious crime, and then commits suicide, it is like bowing down before the victim and lying down next to the one who was wronged. The perpetrator says, "Now I'm here with you, too." You can look at it from this perspective and it's a deep, healing picture.

Albert's mother denied him contact with his real father.

HELLINGER I would suggest that you sit up straight and look around the group. Keep your eyes open.

To group In a panic attack, external contact and keeping your eyes open are very important. When a person closes their eyes, they retreat into imaginary scenes and fantasy pictures.

After a while to Albert Now imagine your real father, when you were small and stood next to him, under his protection.

I'll say a word here about fathers. When children are afraid, their fathers understand that, but the children don't realize that their fathers understand that.

Keep your eyes open. The way to deal with the panic is to keep your mouth opened slightly, keep your eyes open, and lay your hands in your lap with the palms up. Imagine the panic draining away:

- Through your eyes. For example by looking in a friendly manner and bowing your head slightly forward.
- Through breathing – breathing out.
- Through your hands. Imagine a reaching out and up to your father, as a small child, perhaps about four.

Keep your mouth open, that's important, and keep your eyes focussed. It's good if you can look far enough to see your father somewhere and look into his eyes.

After a while You're doing very well now.

EXHAUSTED
Multiple sclerosis

HELLINGER *to Judith, who walks only with great effort using a walker and who can speak only unclearly* What is it?
JUDITH I have multiple sclerosis.
HELLINGER I have a question for you. Can you be helped?
JUDITH Yes.
HELLINGER Wait, wait. You didn't take time to let that into your soul. Can you be helped, or is it exhausted?
JUDITH *shaking her head* No.
HELLINGER It is exhausted.

Long period of silence – Judith is crying.

HELLINGER *to group* I'll explain something about this therapeutic procedure.

When I'm working with someone, I hold an image of that person and where they stand on their path of life. Is the path at an end, or in the middle, or at the beginning? Where is the person at this moment? If I see that this person is standing near the end, then I hold back. If I were to become active, it would be putting myself between the person and the essence of their life. That is something I'm not allowed to do. At this moment, that's something I can't do. The only thing I can do in this moment is to help the person remain collected while looking at the limits, and at death. That's the case here. I can't go any further.

Another long silence.

HELLINGER I'll leave it there, okay?

Judith nods.

To group I'll say something more about the image of the path. Sometimes, when a person comes with an issue, I might notice that the person has forgotten something or left something behind in the past. Then, I can go with the person back to the place where that happened. Perhaps the person needs a blessing from a parent, or perhaps there was some kind of trauma that hasn't been dealt with. Then, I can go back to that place with the person and help him or her to take what is needed, or resolve what is unresolved, and then we return to the present. It's important not to stay in the past!

Sometimes a person reaches some kind of limitation, not a permanent, fixed limitation, but an obstacle along the way. I can help the person to clear away the obstacle so that the way is clear again.

I stay where I am. I don't go on with the patient. I stay at the spot where something is resolved, and the patient goes on alone.

"It's fine"
Intestinal cancer

HELLINGER What is your issue?

GEORGE I know that I've had cancer for three years.

HELLINGER What kind of cancer?

GEORGE Intestinal tumor. I've been operated on repeatedly, and the doctors can't get the malignant cells out of my body.

HELLINGER Are you married?

GEORGE Yes, I have a wife, but no children.

HELLINGER How much time have you got left?

GEORGE *after thinking it over* I think I have less time than most people my age.

HELLINGER Yes. And you're looking forward, not back.

GEORGE *very moved* Yes, sometimes I can see a long way, that's true.

Long silence

GEORGE It's fine.

HELLINGER *to Bea* How do you feel, sitting here next to me?
BEA I'm nervous, but I feel very safe here.

Bea leans against Hellinger and he puts his arm around her.

BEA *after a while* That's nice.
HELLINGER We'll wait a little while.
After a pause, still holding Bea Now, tell me what's the matter with you.
BEA I have had sclerosis for eleven years already. At the moment, I feel like I can't handle it anymore. It's like my reserves are gone, the pot is empty, and a heavy weight is on my shoulders, pressing me down. On the other hand, I think waste my energy on meaningless things.

She has straightened up in the meantime.

HELLINGER Would you like to explain what sclerosis is?
BEA It's a disease of the connective tissue. To begin with, I have too little oxygen. My capabilities are limited because of that, regardless of whether I am working physically or writing something. I also don't acknowledge that.
HELLINGER Set up a constellation with two people, you and your illness.
BEA Does it matter whether I choose a man or a woman to represent the illness?
HELLINGER Choose according to what seems right for you. Then, remain very collected while you place the two in relation to each other.

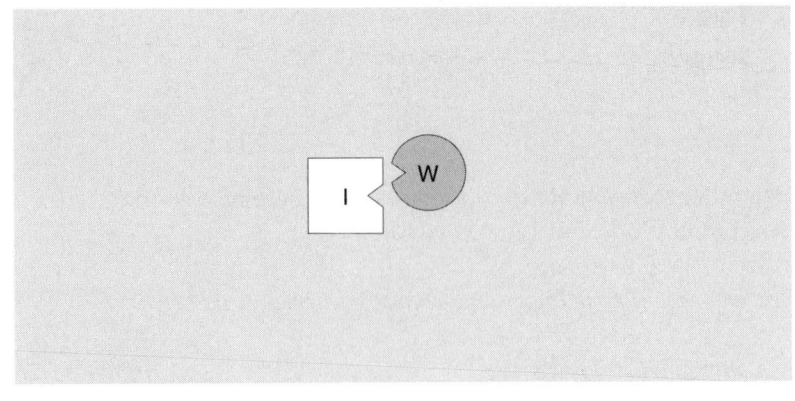

I   Illness
W   Woman (Bea)

After a while, Hellinger turns the representative of the illness more towards Bea's representative and has him put his arm around her. Bea's representative looks down at the floor. After a while, Hellinger raises her head and lays it on the illness' shoulder.

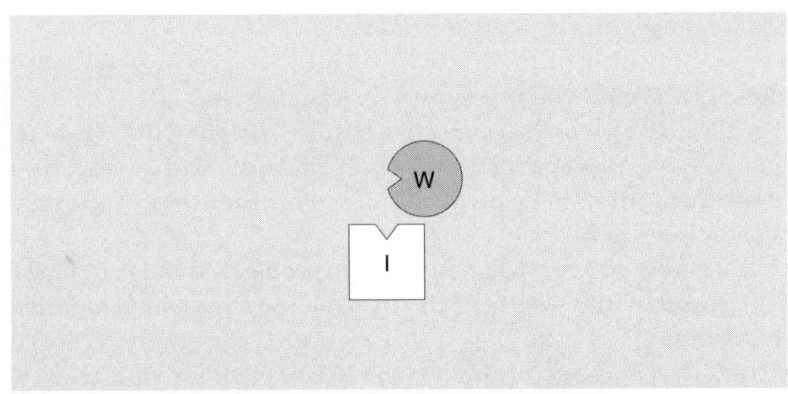

BEA *after a while* That's not right.
HELLINGER Wait a little bit.
After a while, to Bea's representative How are you feeling?
WOMAN At first it was terrible, but now I feel very secure here with this illness. Yes, I feel secure with the illness.
HELLINGER *to the representative of the Illness* And for you?
ILLNESS I'm feeling better and better. At first I couldn't really take on this task, but now it's okay. I feel strong.

After a while, Hellinger puts his arm around Bea again similar to the position of the representative of the illness with Bea's representative. Bea leans against him, but continues to look at the constellation.

HELLINGER *to Bea* How are you doing?
BEA It's getting better.
HELLINGER Yes, exactly.
BEA It's as if I can trust myself.

Hellinger and Bea look at each other.

HELLINGER I think that was it. Okay?
BEA Yes.

HELLINGER *after a while, to group* A while ago someone asked me how I could stand to expose myself to everything in the constellations. He thought that I was at the mercy of something bad. I couldn't answer him, but I thought about it afterwards. What I came up with is that I actually only expose myself to the entirety. Everything has a place and it's all good.

THE SOUL
Celiac disease

HELLINGER What is it?

CLAIRE I have a disease that I had when I was a baby, called celiac disease. It's a reaction to flour. You get diarrhea and feel lousy in general. I can't believe that I haven't had it for 29 years and now I've got it again. But, it's getting better already.

HELLINGER When did it break out again? How long ago?

CLAIRE Last summer. I'm an actress and I was preparing for a film. They said I should lose some weight for this role. I tried to lose weight for about three months to start shooting the film.

HELLINGER I think that's awful.

CLAIRE I didn't lose so much, it was only about three or four kilograms, not ten or anything.

HELLINGER We will set up a constellation with your soul and the film. Okay, go ahead.

CLAIRE My soul and the film?

HELLINGER Your soul and the film, yes.

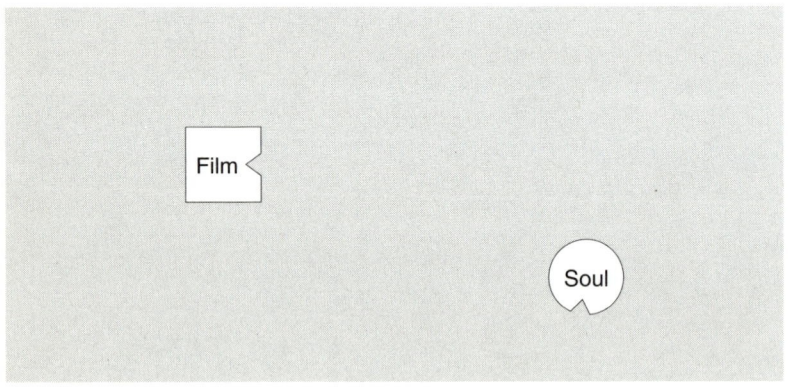

HELLINGER *to Claire, when she has placed the representatives* Now set up a representative for the illness too.

Claire places the illness between the film and her soul. Then she moves it behind her soul.

100

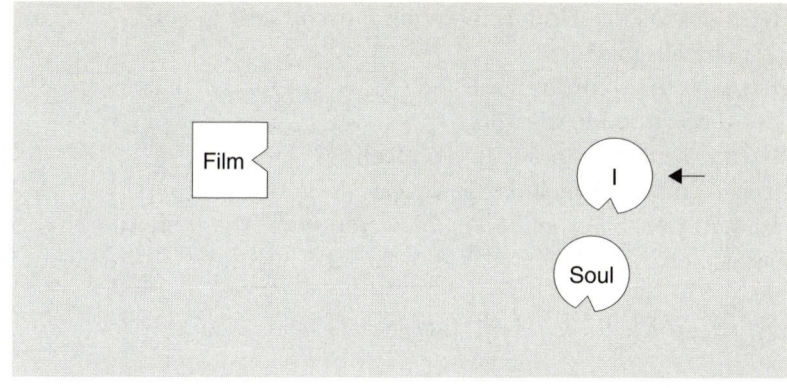

I   Illness

HELLINGER *to soul's representative* How are you feeling?
SOUL At the moment, better. The worst was when she put the film near me. The best was when she had the illness between us. It's also better now, without her.
HELLINGER *to Illness* And you?
ILLNESS I feel sad, and I don't feel well. I feel like I'm going to throw up.
HELLINGER And what's with the film?
FILM I'm a threat to her, I can feel that strongly. Just to be polite, I looked straight ahead instead of directly at her, so she wouldn't feel so threatened.
HELLINGER *to Claire* Take your place in the constellation.

She stands in the position of the soul's representative and Hellinger places the soul next to the film.

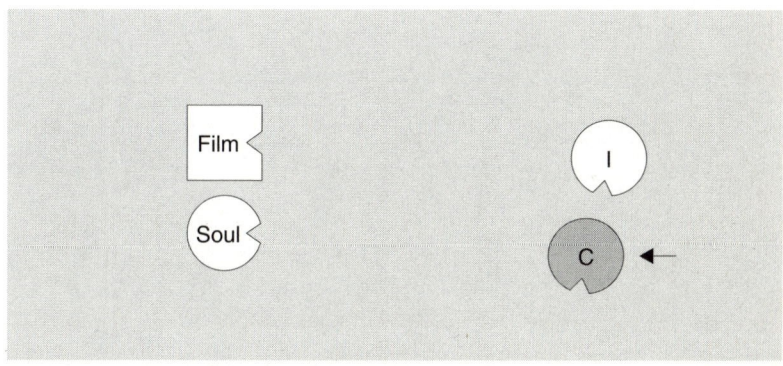

W   Woman (Claire)

101

HELLINGER *to Film* How is it having the soul next to you?
FILM It feels good.
HELLINGER And for the soul?
SOUL Feels good to me, too.
HELLINGER *to Claire* How are you feeling?
CLAIRE I'm a little jealous. *She laughs.*
HELLINGER *to illness and Soul* Now the two of you should change places.

Hellinger places the soul very close behind Claire.

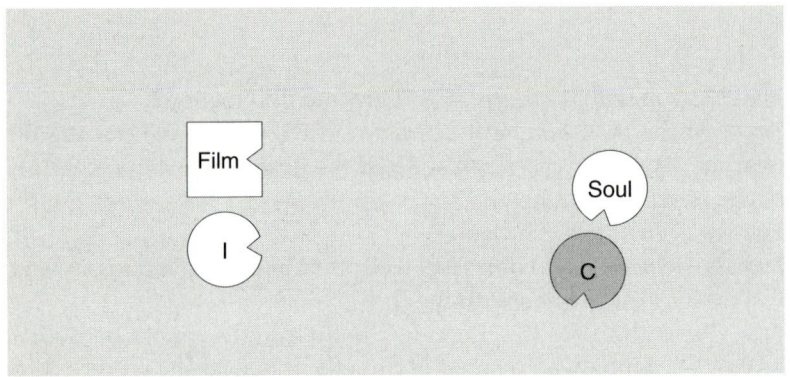

HELLINGER *to Claire* How is that, now?
CLAIRE Now I feel better.

Hellinger places the soul between Claire and the illness and film.

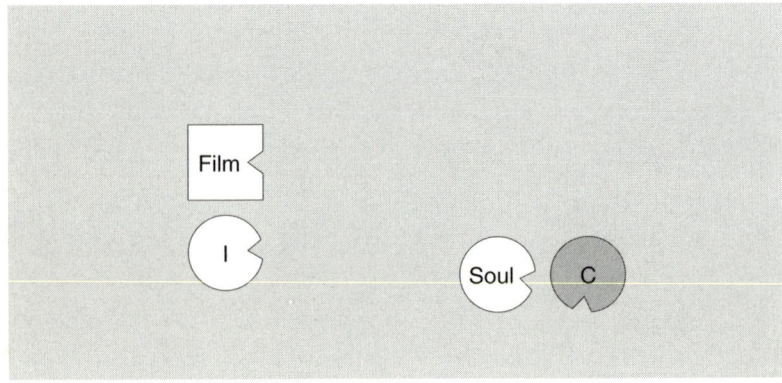

CLAIRE Now I can't see the others any more.
HELLINGER And how is that for you?
CLAIRE Hmm. It's absolutely okay.
HELLINGER How is the soul doing?
SOUL Fine.
HELLINGER The film?
FILM I feel lighter, I've got more air.
ILLNESS I also feel better. It's warmer here and I can see the two standing over there very well.
HELLINGER *to Claire* I don't know what this means, but I'll leave it like that, okay?

Claire nods and laughs.

HELLINGER What's the matter?
CONSTANCE I got skin cancer about six months ago, and I was also burned.
HELLINGER What do you mean?
CONSTANCE I was burned, in a fire.
HELLINGER How old were you then?
CONSTANCE 26.
HELLINGER What happened?
CONSTANCE During Carnival time, I went to a costume party dressed as cotton candy. One of my sisters had on a balloon costume. A woman touched the balloon costume with a lit cigarette and it exploded. Suddenly I was in flames. There was a man who acted quickly. He tore down a curtain and wrapped it around me. I had burns over 70 % of my body and I came close to dying. I was in the hospital for almost a year. That has changed my life with the scars I have.
HELLINGER In what way has it changed your life?
CONSTANCE With men. I couldn't see myself as attractive after that, with these scars all over my body. That happened two weeks before I was supposed to meet my boyfriend in America. Instead, I went into the hospital. Everything in my life has been more difficult, and now I've got skin cancer. Life is really difficult.
HELLINGER Someone said to me a while ago that you can't help someone who is pining away with grief and sorrow. What happened in this fire? You said you came close to dying. What actually happened?
CONSTANCE I didn't go to America to meet my boyfriend, I stayed at home. I have stayed at home ever since, in the family business. That's what happened.
HELLINGER That was pining away. What actually happened?
CONSTANCE Everyone took care of me. All my brothers and sisters took care of me. They all came.
HELLINGER What happens in your soul when you tell that?
CONSTANCE I'm shaking.
HELLINGER Yes, I would be shaking, too.

104

CONSTANCE But I don't know why I'm shaking.

HELLINGER Tell your soul, "You were by my side."

CONSTANCE You were by my side.

HELLINGER How does your soul feel now?

CONSTANCE It's saying, "I'm still with you."

HELLINGER Are you with your soul?

CONSTANCE I think it's hiding.

HELLINGER Yes, your soul hides from you. You didn't honor the gift.

CONSTANCE Gift? That my soul was there when I got burned?

HELLINGER And that you recovered.

CONSTANCE Yes.

HELLINGER How do you feel if you give someone a priceless gift and they throw it away? How does that make you feel?

CONSTANCE It hurts and it makes me sad.

HELLINGER And what is the result?

CONSTANCE Then I pull back and hide.

HELLINGER Yes, then you lose your strength. I have shown you a way.

CONSTANCE A way? To accept the priceless gift?

HELLINGER Have you accepted my gift?

CONSTANCE I wanted something different.

HELLINGER Exactly. That's it. You're looking at me, but who is standing at the door trying to get in?

CONSTANCE Perhaps, my soul?

HELLINGER Yes, your soul. You're cut off from your own soul. What can help you with this cancer?

CONSTANCE I don't know that. I think it's a signal. With the cancer? That's why I wanted to do a family constellation.

HELLINGER Without the soul, nothing happens here.

To group I'd like to say something here about psychosomatic illness. Many people imagine that in a psychosomatic illness, the illness comes from the psyche and the illness will go away if the psyche is brought into order. That's looking at the spirit as something that one uses in order to get well again. But the spirit, or soul, won't stand for being used to achieve health. The soul has purposes that lie far beyond that. What is possible, however, is to win the soul's help. For example, by honoring and respecting the soul and following the spirit's lead, even if this leads through an illness.

Often, psychosomatic illness is regarded as if it had to do with the ego and the body, instead of the soul and the body. That would have to be called ego-somatic illness, and not psychosomatic. When somebody says that an illness is caused by the psyche, and the person should get hold of themselves, it usually means the ego, and not the soul. You have to obey the soul, and it's a humble obedience. This kind of humility heals.

To Constance Did you understand what I said?
CONSTANCE I'm trying to understand it.
HELLINGER I'll give you some time with it, okay?

Constance nods.

HELLINGER *to group* What I just said about people who are ill is also true for therapists, of course. For the therapist to move back from plans and intentions to find a harmony with the soul of the patient. To feel the movement of the soul and move in harmony with this. To help the soul even against the wishes and fantasies of the patient. When the soul is set in motion in this way, then something good comes out of it. Then, you're standing on firm ground and can trust the strength that comes from within.

Clients or patients often come to a therapist and ask for help setting up a family constellation so they'll feel better. That's an appeal to the imagined power of the therapist, as if the therapist really had any power. If a therapist falls into this trap and tries to make something happen, the soul won't go along with it. The work will never succeed.

THE WAY TO THE DEAD
Intestinal cancer

Henry has just finished a family constellation of his present family.

HELLINGER *to Henry* I'm not sure if I can help you get out of this. Come and sit next to me and I'll try something with you. A contemplative exercise. Shall I?
HENRY Yes, please do.
HELLINGER Close your eyes, and breathe calmly and deeply. Bow your head forward slightly. Let it hang.
Imagine you are going towards the dead. … deep down to the dead, whoever they are … including this baby [a previously mentioned aborted child] … until you come to them … then you lie down next to them … until you grow still with them … absolutely still … all the excitement on the earth recedes … and you grow absolutely still … you're one of them … slowly come to rest … until everything is still. Let your head sink deeper down.
After a long pause When you are absolutely still, feel their strength … the strength of the dead … because they are well kept … among them, you're the smallest.
Honor what they give you … each one of them … if you are really with them, something will come to you from them … breathe deeply … now, take it in, with an open mouth, and leave something with the dead, perhaps your pain … and guilt … or something else. Perhaps they will give you pain too, … pain that belongs to you.
A long quiet pause When it is finished, rise slowly back up … and come back.

Henry remains in his bowed position for a long time, then he straightens up slowly and opens his eyes.

HELLINGER *to Henry* Don't talk about this with anyone, okay?

Henry nods and murmurs a thank you.

WE THREE
Muscular dystrophy

HELLINGER *to Angelica* I'll work with you now, if you want.
ANGELICA Yes, I do.
HELLINGER What is wrong with you?
ANGELICA I've had muscular dystrophy since I was born. I inherited it from my mother's family. It first became apparent when I was 15, I'm 31 now. I was an athlete, a swimmer, and my physical ability in sport decreased rapidly. In any case, the disease is progressive, and my strength is ebbing. I'm aware that I want to be okay at whatever level I am. At the moment there's a lot going on in my family. My relationship with my mother is somehow …
HELLINGER Okay, that's enough. Lean against me.

Angelica leans against Hellinger and puts her arm around him. He puts his arm around her.

HELLINGER Who am I representing, now?
ANGELICA My mother.
HELLINGER Yes, exactly. I'm representing your mother.

Hellinger puts both arms around her and holds her tightly. She also puts her arms around him and weeps.

HELLINGER *after a while* What did you call your mother?
ANGELICA Mommy.
HELLINGER Tell her, "Dear Mommy."
ANGELICA Dear Mommy.
HELLINGER "I take it even at this price."
ANGELICA I take it even at this price.
HELLINGER "With love."
ANGELICA With love.
HELLINGER "Dear Mommy."
ANGELICA Dear Mommy.
HELLINGER *after another pause* How do you suppose your mother feels, knowing that you inherited this disease from her?

ANGELICA She feels terrible.
HELLINGER Exactly.

Hellinger releases Angelica from his embrace. She wipes her tears away and breathes deeply.

HELLINGER And how are you doing with this life?
ANGELICA Not too well.

Hellinger chooses a representative and places her facing Angelica.

HELLINGER *to Angelica* This would represent your illness. Tell her, "I take you with my mother."
ANGELICA I have to touch her.

She reaches out her hand to the representative of the disease and smiles at her.

ANGELICA I take you with my mother.
HELLINGER "You two belong together."
ANGELICA You two belong together.

She cries.

HELLINGER Look at her and breathe deeply.
After a while Close your eyes. Take your illness and your mother, both of them now, into your soul.

She closes her eyes and bows her head.

HELLINGER And say, "We three."
ANGELICA *after a long pause* We … we three.
HELLINGER "Are one."
ANGELICA *crying* Are one.
HELLINGER Let the three flow together until they are one unit.

Angelica remains motionless for a long time. Then she lays her head on Hellinger and weeps.

HELLINGER *after a while* How are you feeling now?

ANGELICA Better.

HELLINGER And how is your mother feeling?

ANGELICA Also better.

HELLINGER And your illness?

ANGELICA Also better.

HELLINGER *to representative of the Illness* How are you doing?

ILLNESS I'm doing fine.

HELLINGER *to Angelica* So that's it, your unique fate.

Angelica moves back away from Hellinger and dries her tears. She continues to hold hands with the representative of her illness.

HELLINGER I'll also tell you a little story about life, shall I?

ANGELICA Yes.

HELLINGER Last year I was doing a course in London and there was a woman, about 40 years old, who had had polio as a child. She recovered, but for the three years preceding this workshop she had been getting weaker and was confined to a wheelchair. She was sitting next to me and I told her to imagine herself growing up, completely healthy, like other young girls. Then, I told her to visualize her life as it actually had been, including her disease and weakness. After she had done both, I asked her which life was more precious.

She fought against it for a long time, but then came her tears, and she said, "This life is more precious!"

To Angelica It has a particular greatness and strength. Agreed?

ANGELICA *embracing Hellinger* Yes.

HELLINGER Much love to you.

"DEAR CHILD"
Chronic uterine inflammation

HELLINGER What's going on with you?

SUSANNE I've had a uterine inflammation for the past two years and it just doesn't go away. It just stays at the same degree of disturbance. Sometimes it goes away for a few hours, but it's really always there. It's very limiting, and it bothers me a lot.

HELLINGER Are you married?

SUSANNE No.

HELLINGER Have you got any children?

SUSANNE No.

HELLINGER Did something happen?

SUSANNE Yes, I was pregnant once, but I lost the baby after two months. That was three years ago. Since then, I haven't been in a relationship.

HELLINGER You lost it. Was it a miscarriage?

SUSANNE Yes.

HELLINGER Something happened in your soul. What happened in you?

SUSANNE I didn't want it. I didn't want it just then. I kept thinking, Yes, but not now, please. Later. I've repressed that, but it's still there.

HELLINGER Close your eyes. Imagine the baby and take it back in your lap. Surround it with love.

After a while Breathe deeply with your mouth open. Open your mouth slightly.

After another pause Now, inside yourself, say to the child, "Dear child."

She smiles and nods.

HELLINGER Now let it go, with love. Gently.

She bows her head.

HELLINGER Now pick the baby up and take it into your heart.

after a pause Okay.

SUSANNE Yes.

HELLINGER Good. That's all, then.

HELLINGER *to group* I would like to say something about the dead. In keeping with what we experience and the effects we can observe, it would seem as if the dead remain with us for a while. They are gone in that we can't see them any longer, but they are still present through their effects on us, as if they were still there.

The soul of the family system encompasses the living and the dead equally. That's why the dead require a place in the family. Sometimes people are afraid that the dead will wreak havoc, but, in fact, the opposite is true. The dead are powerful but mild. They attend to the living.

To Susanne Even a dead baby attends to its mother and father. You can see it in the effects.

After a while, however, the dead retreat. If they are respected and honored, if they have been allowed in and allowed to have an effect, then they can pull back when they are finished. Then, you have to let them go. It's an inner movement. We don't know where they go.

To Susanne If you hold on to them, for example, by remembering them too long, the pulling away movement is disturbed. So, after a while, the baby can also leave your heart. Then it will truly be dead and at peace. That's important. But, for a while you need to keep it with you. At least for a year or so. Okay?

SUSANNE Yes.

HELLINGER Good. That's all.

"A LITTLE, BUT NOT TOO MUCH"
A couple who can't decide

HELLINGER What's the issue?

HERMAN It's about our relationship. My problem with this relationship is that Rosa doesn't fully engage. She holds back and doesn't put herself fully into the relationship.

HELLINGER Were either of you in a serious relationship before this one?

HERMAN I was married before, but I've been divorced for 14 years. I've got an 18 year old daughter, who lives with my ex-wife.

HELLINGER A second wife doesn't trust herself to take this man fully. That's simply how it is.

HERMAN But I think that can change. *He laughs.*

HELLINGER I don't know about that. It doesn't come that cheaply.

HERMAN I know that.

HELLINGER *to Rosa* Do you have something to say to this?

ROSA It's not the first time that I've been unable to really enter into a relationship. Actually, I've never done that. From that viewpoint, I'd say it has a lot to do with me. It has a lot to do with my past that I'm afraid to let anyone get too close to me.

HELLINGER You're not marriage-able, or something like that?

ROSA You could say that.

HELLINGER Have you got children?

HERMAN No.

ROSA We're also not married. Herman would like to get married. I'm too afraid, and even had a disc go out in my back when we were going to get engaged. That was the end for a while. *Both laugh.*

HELLINGER I think perhaps that's the best solution. A little, but not too much.

ROSA That's not very satisfying over the long haul.

HELLINGER If it weren't satisfactory, it would have changed. It's the best thing possible for the two of you.

They both look at each other very seriously for a long time.

HELLINGER Now there's a seriousness in this. I'll leave it right there.

To group Now we're standing on firm ground. They are grounded, and I'm grounded too. If you're on the ground, you can walk, but not in the clouds.

Rudolph My wife is jealous.

Hellinger Jealousy means the jealous one wants to get rid of the partner. Is that so?

Ulrike No, that's not so.

Hellinger I'm not so sure. Jealousy usually wants the opposite of what it seems to want. Not to hold on to the partner, but to get rid of him. And jealousy is an infallible way to achieve that. Instead of leaving the partner, it forces the partner to leave. That's really the function of jealousy. That's a comfort for everyone who suffers from jealousy.

Ulrike I'm speechless. For me, jealousy has been more of a problem that has to do with my sense of self-worth, that I always have to compare myself to someone else.

Hellinger What does a man love in a woman besides the woman-being. What does a woman love in a man except the man-being? They both love the soul, and the soul is incomparable. Agreed?

Ulrike Yes.

Rudolph Yes.

Hellinger *as they look into each other's eyes* Where can you see the soul? In the eyes. When you look into each other's eyes, you see nothing else.

"YES, GLADLY"
Choosing one another and a child

HELLINGER What is it?

FELICITY We're expecting a baby in about three weeks. This pregnancy has had a lot more downs than ups, and now there's just a feeling that I can't have this baby. I'm not ready. In the past couple of days, I've become aware of how much baggage we're still carrying from our families of origin. My sense of being a mother is very shaped by my experiences with my family.

HELLINGER I don't need so many details. We can see the essentials. Are you married?

FELICITY No.

HELLINGER Why not?

FELICITY Up till now I haven't wanted to think about getting married, and so I haven't.

HELLINGER And what does the child want? Can you imagine?

FELICITY A family.

HELLINGER Yes, exactly. These days it's not so 'in' to get married. Do you know why? There's really only one reason. Practically speaking, there's only one reason – the desire to extend adolescence.

FELICITY Yes, there's something to that.

HELLINGER But when you have a baby, adolescence is over.

FELICITY That's an issue, I think.

HELLINGER What does the man have to say here?

MANUEL I've got a problem with this baby, the closer it comes. I'm aware that at the moment, I just can't find a place for this child.

HELLINGER You're in competition with the baby.

MANUEL I don't see that.

HELLINGER Let's do a very simple exercise.

Hellinger places Felicity in the middle, with Manuel behind her. He has Manuel put his hands on her shoulders. Then, he has Felicity lean back against Manuel.

116

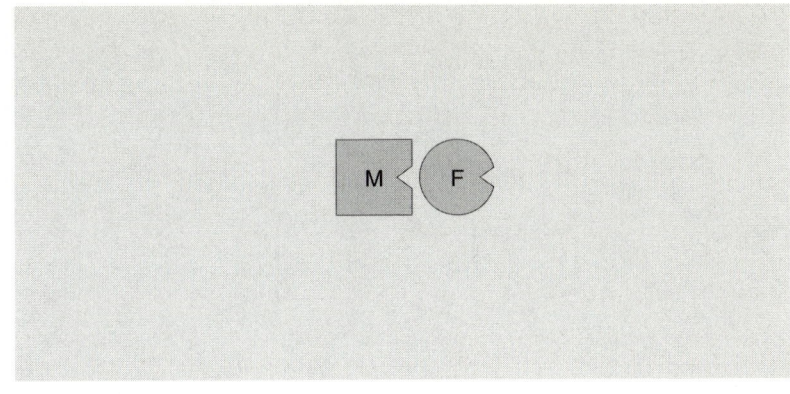

M   **Man (Manuel)**
W   **Woman (Felicity)**

After a while, Hellinger chooses a representative for Manuel's father and places him behind Manuel, with his hands on Manuel's shoulders.

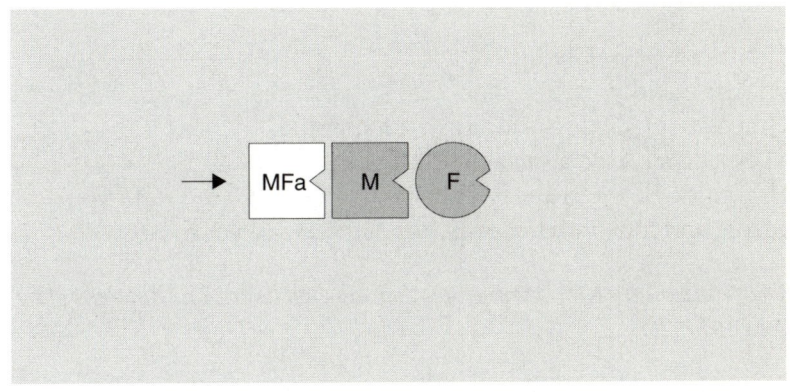

MF   Man's father

After another pause, Hellinger bows Manuel's head forward so that he is touching Felicity's head. Somewhat later, he turns Felicity towards Manuel. They embrace. Felicity lays her head on Manuel's chest.

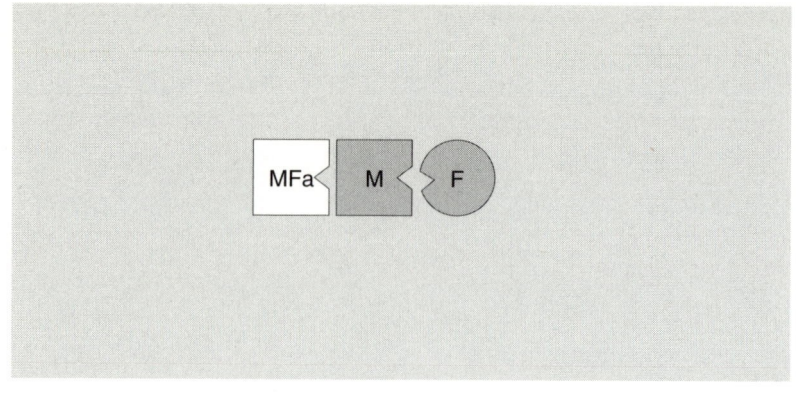

Hellinger *to Manuel and Felicity* Look each other in the eye.
To Manuel Tell her, if you can, "Yes." But you have to look into her eyes as you say it.
Manuel *after some hesitation* Yes.
Hellinger *to Felicity* You say it too.
Felicity Yes.
Hellinger Say, "Gladly."
Felicity Gladly.
Hellinger *to Manuel* You say that to her too.
Manuel *after some hesitation* Gladly.
Hellinger Say it in a way that she'll believe it. Wait until your soul agrees and look into her eyes. You have to say yes to two.

The representative for Manuel's father lays his hands on Manuel's shoulders again.

Manuel *after a while in a firm voice* Yes, gladly.
Hellinger That was good.
To Felicity Is that okay ? *She nods.* You have to look at him. You say it too. "Yes, gladly."
Felicity Yes, gladly.
Hellinger *after a while, as they continue looking at each other* Whatever else there is from your families of origin, that belongs in another context. This, here, is what's essential. You two are the essential people here.
To Manuel, who is wiping away his tears Is that okay for you?
Manuel Yes. Somehow it was clear to me that all this had something

118

to do with my father. He died very suddenly, and since then things haven't been so good between us. *He is very emotional.*

HELLINGER Stand next to your wife, facing your father.

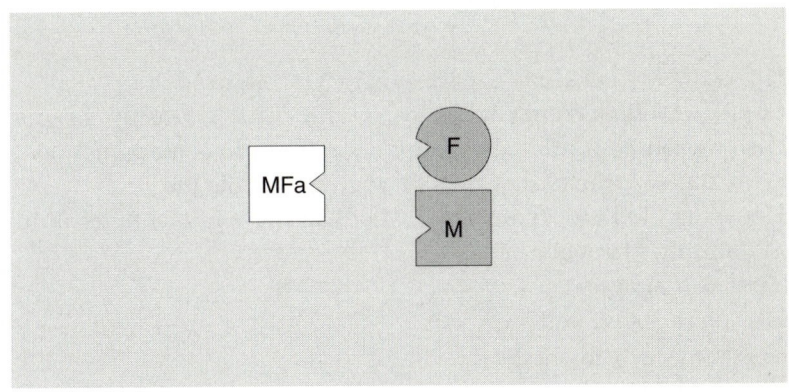

As Manuel stands next to Felicity, he puts his arm around her and strokes her.

HELLINGER *to Manuel* Say to your father, "Look kindly on us and on our child."

MANUEL Look kindly on us and on our child.

HELLINGER "See, it goes on."

MANUEL See, it goes on.

MANUEL'S FATHER That I do gladly.

HELLINGER *to Manuel* Okay?

MANUEL Yes.

HELLINGER *to Felicity* Is that good for you?

FELICITY Yes.

HELLINGER All the best to both of you and your child.

"WHAT'S GOOD CAN GET BETTER"
A couple finds a new beginning

HELLINGER *to Conrad and Cecilia* What's your issue?
CONRAD Well, of course it has to do with our relationship. I experience myself as continually under a strain to do something good. I think this is a thread that runs through my whole life.
HELLINGER Tell her, "I am good." Look at her while you say it. Just say, simply, "I am good."
CONRAD I am good.
HELLINGER "And you are good."
CONRAD And you are good.
HELLINGER *to Cecilia* You tell him, too.
CECILIA You are good, and I am good, too.

They both laugh.

HELLINGER *to Conrad* With this goodness, it's the same as with luck. There's a secret. Do you know what it is? It can get better.
CECILIA Goodness?
HELLINGER Yes, what's good can get better. And it's best together.
A relationship lives and develops through confirmation of one another "That was nice." – "I liked that" – "That suits you." – "You've done well." – "That tasted nice." I'm talking about very simple things. And when something doesn't please you, you can wonder what might be good in that, too.

There's another secret, how to secure and develop your relationship. A river lives from its source. That's where it springs from and that's where it becomes a river. When things get difficult, you go back to the source - the first meeting, for example. When you visualize that, you may find a glow in your eyes and on your face.

There's another secret for building your relationship. When something has gone wrong, or where there have been problems, you put it aside and never speak of it again. It simply is never spoken of, and never thought about. It's possible to do that. The skilled, they can do that.
CONRAD *to Hellinger* She just asked me if we can do that. I told her we'll manage it.

120

HELLINGER   Good. There's another secret for good relationships. It goes together with what I just said. You grant each other a fresh start. *To Conrad* Anything else?

CONRAD   Would you ask her?

HELLINGER *to Cecilia* Anything else?

CECILIA   No, that was very enlightening.

HELLINGER   Are you satisfied, or was there something else that needed attention?

CECILIA   Actually, that was enough.

CONRAD   Yes, it's enough.

HELLINGER   I think so, too. An experienced couple like you can do the rest yourselves.

Both laugh.

"I LET YOU GO, WITH LOVE"
Grieving for two deceased wives

HELLINGER What's going on with you two?

LEO We've been together for three and a half years, and have lived together for two and a half years. For the past year, we've been discovering, almost daily, enormous differences between us. Lately we've been questioning whether it makes any sense to even try to work out these differences.

HELLINGER What happened before? There must have been something.

LEO I had two serious relationships before this one, and they both ended with the death of the woman.

HELLINGER What did they die of?

LEO The first one died within three days of a brain hemorrhage. I wasn't married to her. The second woman, who I was married to, died in a car accident while we were on holiday in Namibia.

HELLINGER Who was driving?

LEO Someone else. There were seven of us, and another person in the group was at the wheel. We had an accident and it was in the middle of the desert, so it was an hour and a half before we got any help. Of course I've asked myself over and over how much of those experiences I'm bringing into this relationship.

HELLINGER Choose two representatives for the two women who died, and a representative for the driver of the car.

When Leo has chosen representatives, Hellinger sets up the representatives in relation to Leo.

122

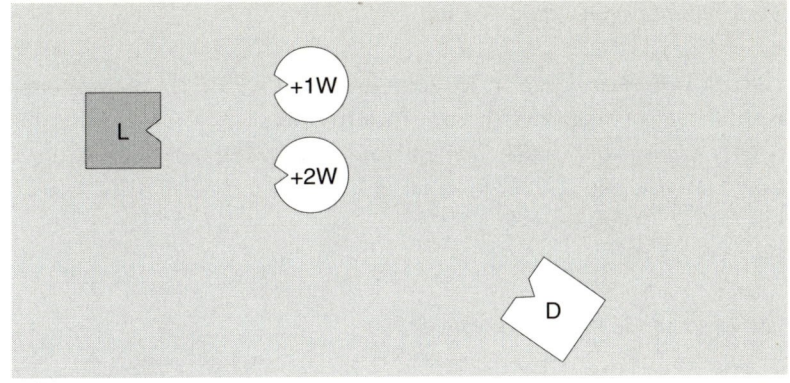

M   **Man (Leo)**
+1W   First wife, died of a brain hemorrhage
+2W   Second wife, died in a car accident
D   Driver of the car

HELLINGER I'll wait for a bit to see how you're doing.
After a while, to Leo Go over to your second wife and hold her. Hold her tightly, just however it seems right to you.

He goes to her and they embrace warmly for a long time. Then they release their embrace and look deeply at each other. Afterwards, they embrace again and again look into each other's eyes.

HELLINGER *to Leo* Stand next to her and put your arm around her.

He stands next to her, and they put their arms around each other.

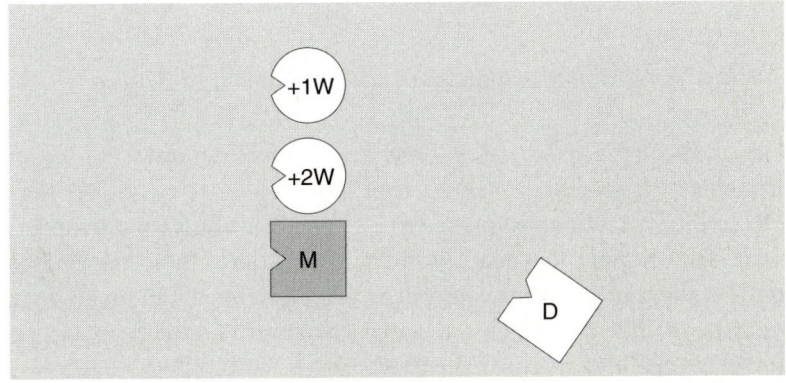

They embrace again, emotionally.

HELLINGER *to Leo* Give in to your impulse, whatever movement is right. Breathe deeply with your mouth open.
After a while as they finish their embrace, to Leo Tell her, "I let you go."
LEO I let you go.
HELLINGER "With love."
LEO With love.

Leo sobs and the two embrace again.

HELLINGER Give in to the pain. "I let you go, with love."

After a long while, they release each other.

HELLINGER Now, stand between the two women and put an arm around each of them.

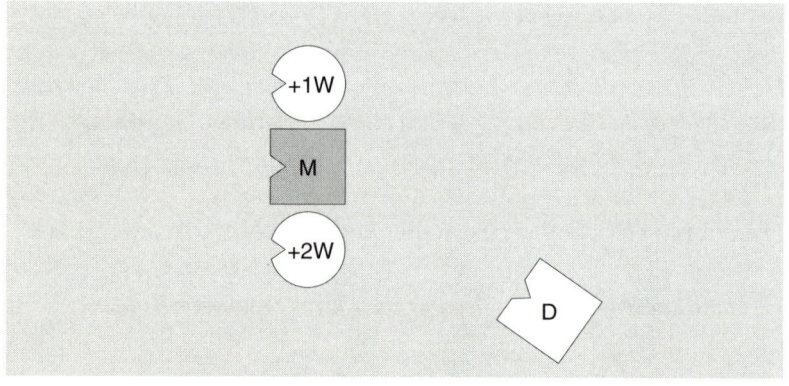

All three put their arms around each other and look at each other.

HELLINGER *after a while, to Leo* How are you feeling, now?
LEO *(sighs)* Lighter.
HELLINGER You weren't finished grieving. Now you've made up a bit of it. That honors the dead women. Your grief honors them. Hold both of them in your heart and then, after a while, let them go out of your heart. The dead aren't at peace if we don't let them go. Do you have any feelings towards the driver?

LEO *after a hesitation* Forgiveness.

HELLINGER Forgiveness isn't allowed. But you can let him stand there with no accusations.

LEO Yes.

HELLINGER That's it. Just let him be without accusations. Okay?

LEO Yes.

HELLINGER *to driver of car* How are you doing?

DRIVER I'd like to move away a bit.

HELLINGER Do it.

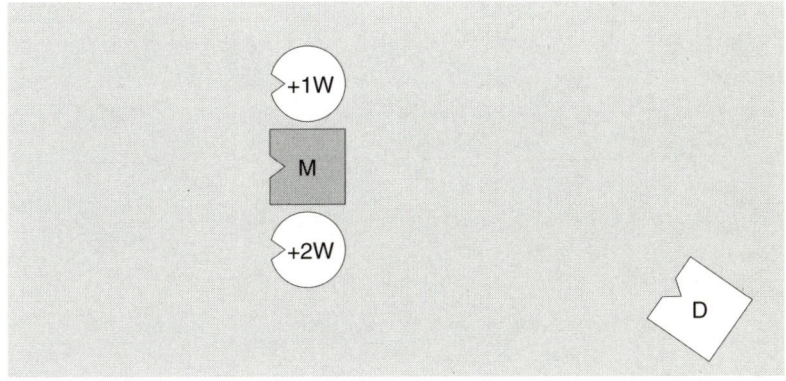

HELLINGER *to group* Any accusations would further hinder the grief process.

To deceased second wife How are you feeling now?

SECOND WIFE I'm doing well now. Before it wasn't good at all. There was just a huge emotional tie to him. Now it's fine.

HELLINGER *to Leo* She wasn't free to go, because you hadn't grieved completely. That happened here.

To deceased first wife And for you now?

FIRST WIFE Now it's fine for me too.

HELLINGER Good. That was it.

Leo sits down next to Helena again.

HELLINGER *to Helena* Do you understand him better now?

HELENA Some things came out that I've felt for a long time, with that grieving. I've felt for a long time that something was missing.

HELLINGER You need to see him with the dead women. Then, you can understand him better and you can replace the dead women.

125

Leo and Helena look at each other and smile. Leo puts his arm around her and she puts a hand on his leg.

HELLINGER *to Helena* Take the love from them. That's a good way.
To Leo and Helena Go ahead and look at each other. This is no first love, but a mature love. That has a different quality to it.

Both nod.

HELLINGER Good, we'll leave it there.

If we look at the effects, it would appear that the dead leave us slowly, as if they would like to stay close by for a while. The dead who are not honored or grieved for, or who are simply forgotten, seem to stay around an especially long time. Also, when the dead are feared, or the survivors want nothing to do with them, the effects from the dead may continue for a very long time.

Grieving can be accomplished by going into the pain and honoring and paying respect to the dead through this pain. When the dead are mourned and honored, they retreat. Then life is finished for them and they can be dead.

Rilke wrote a poem about Orpheus, Eurydice, and Hermes. In the poem, he says of Eurydice, "All inwardness. And replete with her deadness." Being dead is a completion. If we have this image of the dead, then we behave differently. The same holds true for those who die young, even for children who die at birth. We may imagine that they have missed out on something. What could they have missed? The essence is before and after. We spring into life out of that essential and we sink out of life back into it.

When we allow the dead to go, they are benevolent towards us, without getting in our way, without any special effort on our part. A long mourning holds the dead back, even when they want to go, and that is as bad for the living as for the dead. You will often see an extended mourning in cases where the survivor owes the dead person something and has not acknowledged it.

Love doesn't demand a long mourning. Freud commented on President Wilson's re-marriage a year after his wife's death, that it was a sign of his love for his first wife. When a person has loved and mourned, life can go on and the beloved dead will agree to that.

"DO SOMETHING!"
Aortic valve stenosis

HELLINGER *to Cordelia* What is it?

CORDELIA I have an aortic valve stenosis and I don't want an opera-tion. There's no sensible reason, except that I feel resistant to the idea. If I don't have the operation, then, according to the doctors, my heart isn't good for much longer.

HELLINGER Set up a constellation with two representatives.

CORDELIA Two people?

HELLINGER Yes, you and your heart.

When she has chosen the representatives Now place them in relation to each other.

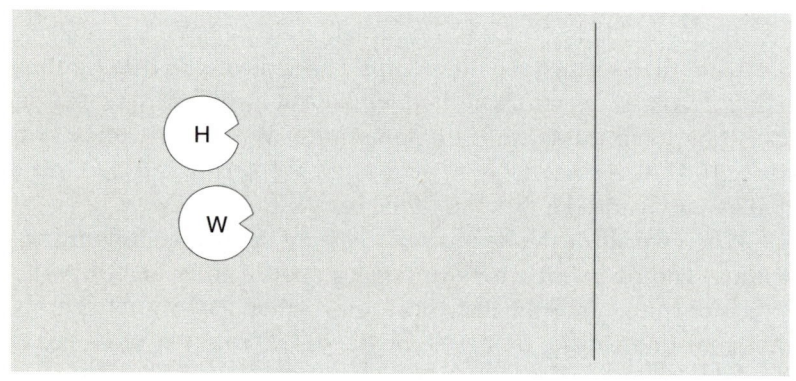

| H | Heart |
| **W** | **Woman (Cordelia)** |

HELLINGER *to the two representatives* I'm not going to say anything. I'll leave you in charge of your own movements. Give in to your im-pulses.

The representative of Cordelia's heart becomes very agitated, clutches her own heart, runs up and down the stage and finally, out the door. Cordelia also clutches her heart.

128

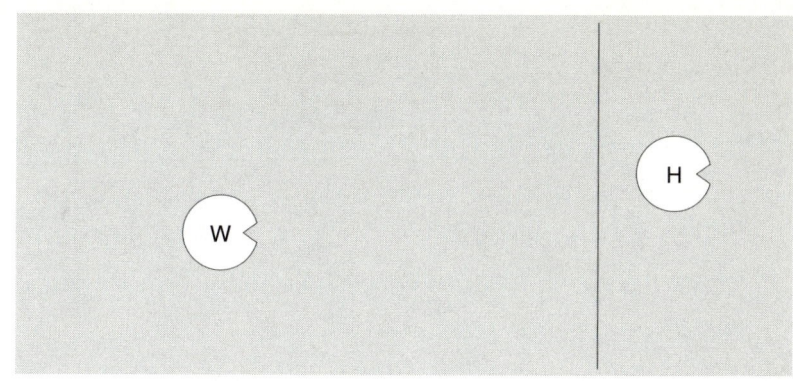

HELLINGER *to Cordelia's representative, as she looks uncertainly towards the door through which her heart has disappeared* Well, do something! Get going! Do something!

She runs through the door after the heart. There is laughter in the audience.

HELLINGER *to group* No, no. You have to stay quiet. This is a matter of life or death.

Hellinger watches through the open door as Cordelia's representative occupies herself with the representative of the heart.

After a while, to Cordelia Go over and watch what's happening.
To group Her representative is stroking the heart and is trying to take care of it. I can see them from here.

Cordelia brings the two representatives back in and stands with them in front of Hellinger.

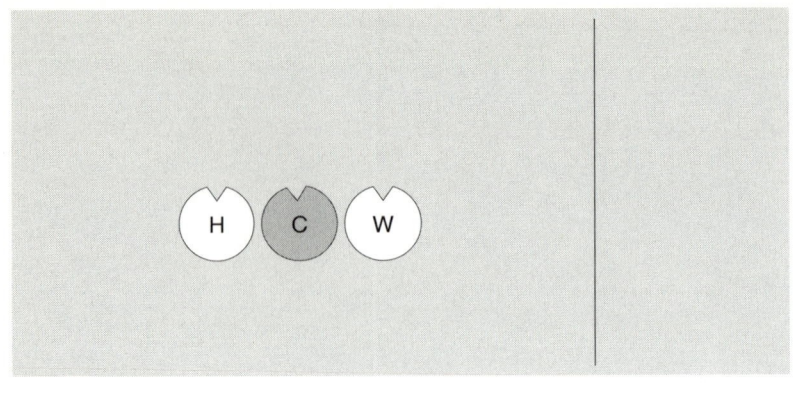

C   Cordelia

CORDELIA I find this rather strange, what's happened here.
HELLINGER What are you going to do?
CORDELIA I'm going to hold them together.
HELLINGER And how are you going to do that?
CORDELIA Yeah, well they've got to stay together, somehow.
HELLINGER What does that mean in practice?
CORDELIA This heart has to feel okay with me.
HELLINGER How can it?
CORDELIA I've got to provide the right conditions.
HELLINGER What's the right condition to provide first?
CORDELIA I have to have the operation.
HELLINGER Yes, you have to have the operation. Okay, that's all.

To group It's very strange what happens sometimes. I didn't do anything except put the arrow in the bow. It shot itself and took off. Things like that can happen when you leave it up to the process and if the therapist follows only what actually comes from the movements.

I had a rather peculiar experience recently. In January I held a course for cancer patients for the Austrian Oncology Society. There was a woman there who was very seriously ill with cancer. I worked with her but nothing happened, and I had to break off the work. She was totally cut off and hidden. The following day she said that she absolutely had to do something because she was having really terrible thoughts. I asked her to come up again. She said she had suddenly remembered that she had had two abortions. As she said this,

130

she was shaking all over. Then she said that the really peculiar thing that had happened was that when she was operated on for the cancer, and woke up from the anesthetic, her adult daughter came in to see her and said, "Mama, at home two children were screaming. I've brought them with me." And the daughter symbolically placed two children on her shoulders. They were the aborted babies. The daughter knew nothing about the abortions, however.

Things have effects when you're able to reach this level. It's eerie what happens sometimes. The woman I was telling you about was able to take these two children into her heart, and suddenly she had vitality. She was thriving, and could set up her family constellation.

"I'll come soon"
Agreeing to death

HELLINGER You are seriously ill?
MATHILDA Two and a half years ago my right breast was removed. I recovered well over the next year and a half and thought I had made it. Nine months ago, there was a recurrence in the same place. I feel shattered. Recently, I followed the advice to have all my teeth pulled out, and because of that I could hardly eat. I now weigh only 40 kilograms. I'm just skin and bones. *She is very emotional.*
HELLINGER Close your eyes, and bow your head slightly. Inside yourself, say, "Yes."
As she turns her head towards him Wait. We have time. Let this yes spread through your body until it has reached every corner, the breast and the heart, the whole soul "Yes!" and death, too ... until there's peace. Imagine all the dead from your family, and tell them, "I'll come soon, with love."

After a while she bows her head.

HELLINGER That's the movement. Stay with that movement. That's the surrender.

She bows her head lower.

HELLINGER Yes, go with the movement, simply.
After a while How are you feeling now?
MATHILDA Calmer.
HELLINGER Good. That's it.
As she turns towards him Can we leave it there?
MATHILDA *hesitates* Was that all?
HELLINGER It was the most major.
MATHILDA That I'm going to die soon?
HELLINGER That you look at it and agree to it.
After a while, she nods I'll show you something more, okay? *She nods.*
I'll choose a representative for death. Is death a man or a woman?

MATHILDA Many. My mother, my father, my natural father, my brother, a son, my grandparents, everyone. I only have my children still.

HELLINGER *to group* She changed it around, and I'll follow her just as she has said it.

Hellinger chooses seven representatives for Mathilda's dead family members and places them standing next to one another. He then asks Mathilda's therapist to represent Mathilda in the constellation, and stands her next to the dead.

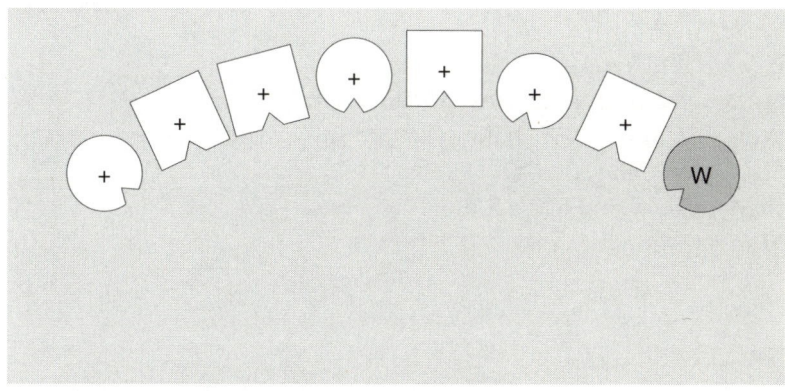

+ the dead members of Mathilda's family
W Woman (Mathilda)

HELLINGER *to Mathilda's representative* How are you feeling there.

WOMAN *crying* It's unbearably sad here.

HELLINGER Look at the dead and tell them, "I'll come, too."

WOMAN *crying* I'll come, too.

HELLINGER *to the dead family members* Look over here, all of you.

WOMAN I'll come, too. I feel such a resistance. In fact, I don't want to.

After a while, Hellinger presents Mathilda's representative to the dead and has them form a circle around her.

The dead reach out to her and touch her.

HELLINGER *to Mathilda's representative* Open your eyes. Look around you with your eyes open and say, "I'll come soon."

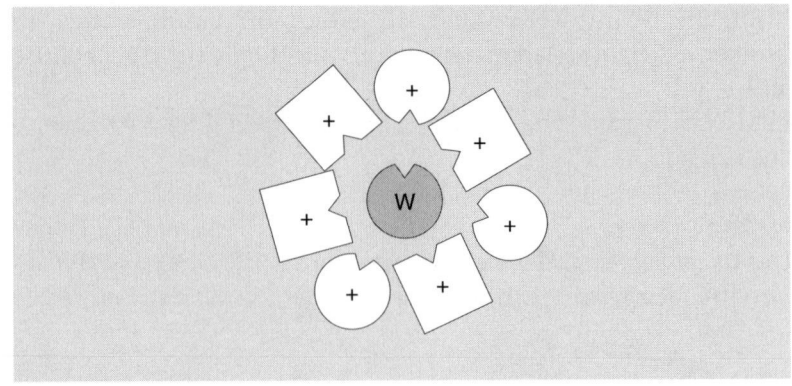

WOMAN I'll come soon. *She sighs.*
HELLINGER *after a while* How are you feeling, now?
WOMAN Calmer. The shaking has stopped. I can come now.
HELLINGER Okay, that's it.
To Mathilda Can I leave it there?
MATHILDA *nodding* Yes.

HELLINGER *to Hans, who is in a wheelchair* You told me you had polio?
HANS Yes.
HELLINGER How old were you?
HANS It was just before my second birthday.
HELLINGER How do you get along with your illness?
HANS I'm at a point now where I'm aware that I can't settle down in my life. The impairments are a constant challenge for me to manage and there's also a lot of familial chaos.
HELLINGER What do you mean by familial?
HANS Familial means that my second wife just moved out. Our separation is somewhat open. I've been living alone for a couple of weeks. As I look back, I can see that there was a lot going on below the surface.
HELLINGER You were married before?
HANS Yes.
HELLINGER For how long?
HANS In the first relationship, for 17 years.
HELLINGER Have you got any children?
HANS Yes.
HELLINGER How many?
HANS Seven. Four from the first marriage and three from the second.
HELLINGER Do you respect your wives?
HANS The first more than the second.
HELLINGER Why did the first marriage break up?
HANS That's difficult to say. After 30 years of stability following the polio, there was a collapse, which I really only recognized in hindsight about five or six years later. In the course of the growth of the first family, demands emerged which led me to flee.
HELLINGER Why did your first wife marry a handicapped man?
HANS That's difficult to say. She had always wanted to be a nurse, and I suppose she had a helping instinct.
HELLINGER Do you respect her?
HANS Yes.
HELLINGER No.

After a while, to a participant sitting nearby The way he talked about her, did he respect her?

PARTICIPANT No.

HELLINGER "She had a helping instinct!"

After a while I have a radical view of this which is: When someone has a particularly difficult fate, such as polio, then that person cannot burden another with this fate. If another declares themselves willing to share the burden, that is extraordinarily special, and can only be accepted with humility and gratitude.

After another pause The one who takes more than he gives is the one who has to leave. It is a truly un-meetable demand which is unbearable.

HANS Could you repeat that?

HELLINGER When there's an inequality in a relationship, where one partner has to give more than he or she receives – for example in marrying someone with a handicap, it is always the case, that the handicapped partner receives more than he or she can give – then the partner who takes more is forced to leave, because it's unbearable. That is, unless that partner is very humble. Then it's possible to take and to stay because the special gift is acknowledged. Does that make any sense to you?

HANS Yes, that makes sense.

HELLINGER There's still something to be made up in relation to your first wife, and that's a deep respect. You also have to communicate to your children that you have a deep respect for your first wife. And then, exactly the same thing with your second wife. I'll leave you with that for now. Is that okay with you?

HANS That's fine.

PARTICIPANT I'd like to know more about the nature of this disrespect.

HELLINGER I can tell you how to get rid of it.

PARTICIPANT I just heard that.

HELLINGER It is a slight movement of the head, from head held high to a bowed head. Like this.

PARTICIPANT Thank you.

136

"THIS IS MY PLACE"
Multiple ailments

HELLINGER What is your issue?

MELANIE I've had a lot of diseases, ever since I was a child, and they're getting worse.

HELLINGER What sort of disease?

MELANIE Immune system defects, later, various accidents, vertebral fractures in my back, muscular dystrophy, and now cancer.

HELLINGER What kind of cancer?

MELANIE Breast cancer. The worst thing for me is that I just can't feel any self-worth, or self-respect. Another major theme for me, even as a child, has been pain – physical pain. I can't do anything for myself.

HELLINGER Are you married?

MELANIE Many years ago I was married for three years.

HELLINGER Have you got any children?

MELANIE No, that wasn't possible at that time because of the back problem.

HELLINGER Then we'll set up a constellation of your family of origin. Who belongs to your family?

MELANIE Father, mother, brother.

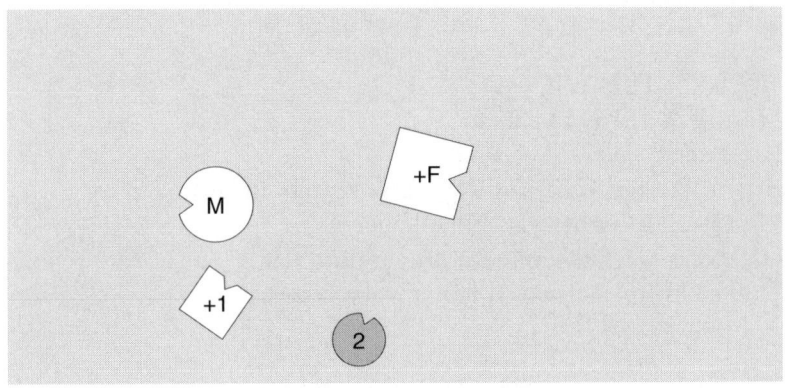

+F Father, killed in the war when Melanie was nine
M   Mother
+1 First Child, a son, had polio
2   Second Child, a daughter (Melanie)

HELLINGER Were your parents divorced?

MELANIE No, my father died very young.

HELLINGER How old were you then?

MELANIE I was three when he went off to war. I hadn't really seen much of him at that point. Then, he was killed when I was nine.

HELLINGER Your mother never re-married?

MELANIE No, she attempted suicide. Before he died, my brother was completely paralyzed from polio.

HELLINGER That's a lot. This family has had a very difficult fate.
To mother's representative What's going on with you?

MOTHER I can't stand up.

Hellinger moves her next to her husband.

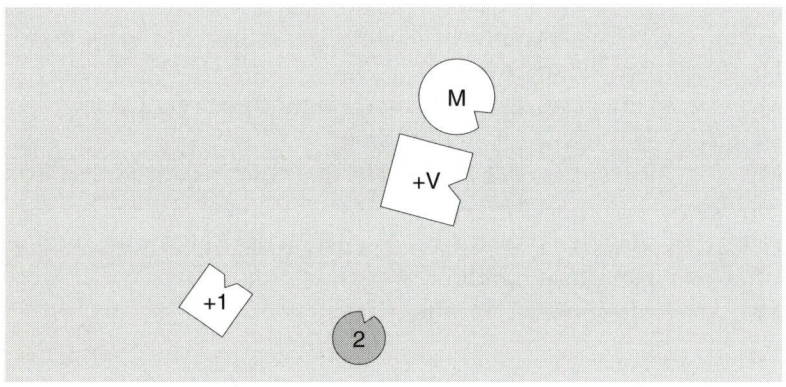

HELLINGER How is it, now?

MOTHER It's okay like that.

HELLINGER *to father* And you?

FATHER Strength and sadness, both. I can hold her.

MOTHER *sighs* Otherwise I'll fall over.

HELLINGER *to father* Put your arm around her.
To son Go and stand next to her, very close to her.

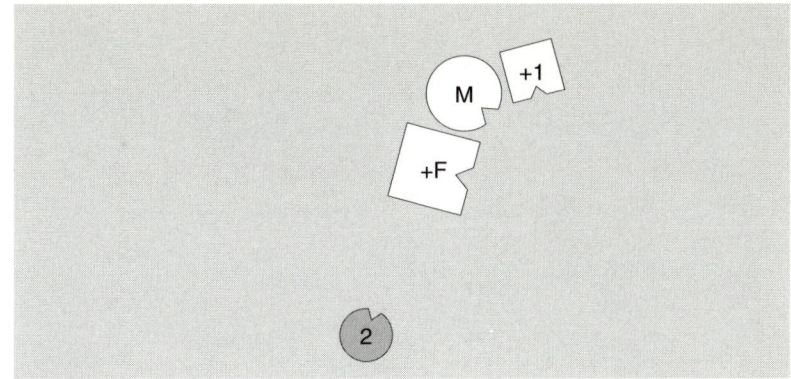

HELLINGER *to Melanie's representative* How are you doing?
SECOND CHILD I have a lot of pain in my back and I want to cry, but
nothing comes out. Everything is all blocked up.
HELLINGER Go and stand next to your brother and put your arm
around him.

*She puts her arm around him and he puts his around her. Her father looks at
her.*

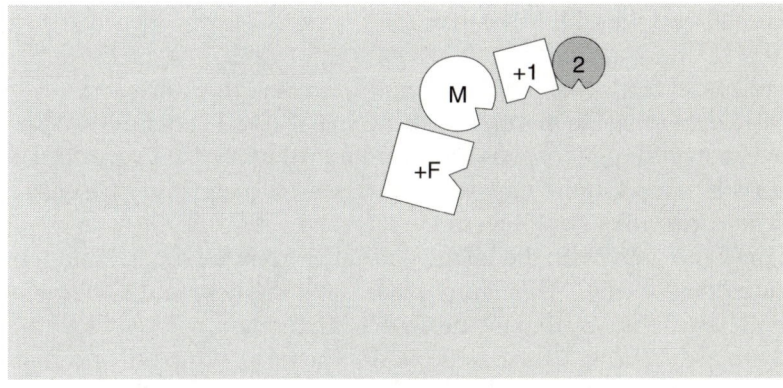

HELLINGER All of you move together in an embrace.

They cluster in a group embrace and lay their heads together.

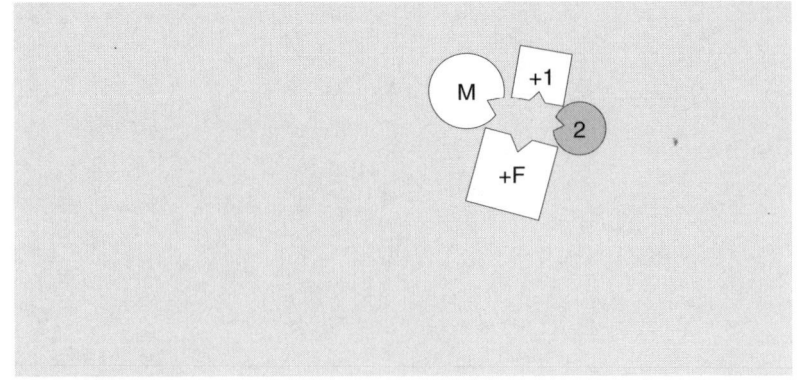

HELLINGER *after a while* How is it now?

FIRST CHILD *sighing* The sadness is still there, even though this is very pleasant. But there's also something very heavy and difficult here.

MOTHER In spite of everything, I have a sense of deep calm about it all. This is right.

FIRST CHILD It also feels right to me for us all to be together.

SECOND CHILD I got very calm, and then, once I felt quiet, there was a connection to all the others. I could feel my own heart and theirs, too. There's a lovely feeling of warmth.

HELLINGER Okay, I'll leave that.

HELLINGER *to Melanie* This is a connection that gives strength.

MELANIE I forgot to mention earlier that I also feel very guilty. Whenever something more goes wrong with my health, I am very hard on myself. I don't know why these illnesses are there, and my sense of self-worth sinks even lower.

HELLINGER Stay with the image that came from the constellation. Inside yourself say, "This is my place. I belong here and I'm staying with you." Just say that inside. In this family there is a lot of love and there are no accusations, none at all. There is deep pain, and that's all. If there's a place made, then peace can flow in. Is that okay for you?

Melanie cries.

HELLINGER Close your eyes … breathe deeply … yes, that's it … stay like that … breathe deeply, that's it … breathe with your mouth open … yes, that's it … lean against me, like this.

Melanie lays her head on Hellinger's shoulder. He puts his arm around her. She cries for a long time.

MELANIE *sitting up* I feel like I don't have to fight any more. I've been fighting all my life.

HELLINGER Now peace is possible, okay?

MELANIE Thank you very much, thank you.

HELLINGER *to group* In the soul there's an attraction towards the dead and towards dying; this is a gentle, deep movement. The movement of our entire life is one that heads back towards that source we sprang from. From there, where life arose, there's a pull on this life to return. You could see it clearly here, that very deep, gentle movement. How much greater this is than what we usually call happiness. Going with this movement brings a person into harmony with everything that is, whatever it is.

To Melanie Sometimes, out of that movement, there's a sense of a fresh wind picking you up. Then, a person may follow the movement prematurely, before it's really time, and that's not a good thing. It has to be exactly right.

MELANIE Otherwise they die too early.

HELLINGER I see you've felt this fresh breeze. Okay.

HELLINGER *to Gertrude* We've worked together before?

GERTRUDE Yes, a year and a half ago.

HELLINGER And it didn't help?

GERTRUDE Oh, yes, it did.

HELLINGER Why are you here again?

GERTRUDE Because life goes on, and I have some more questions.

HELLINGER What is it?

GERTRUDE I have had diabetes since I was 13. I have a daughter who is 10 who is severely handicapped. She is spastic. I had several interrupted pregnancies because in my family, on my mother's side, there's a genetic illness. My mother, my grandmother, and three of my aunts have died, and two of my siblings are also dying. My elder sister was fatally injured in a car accident shortly before my mother died. I don't know where to go from here. I feel like I'm facing a huge wall, a blockade, and I feel guilty about everything.

HELLINGER Are you affected by this genetic disease?

GERTRUDE No.

HELLINGER What disease is it?

GERTRUDE Huntington's Chorea.

HELLINGER What did we do the last time?

GERTRUDE You brought in all the dead relatives in the family, and my brother who is already ill. At that point, though, my sister wasn't there – the one who died as a result of the accident. I bowed to all of them, together with my daughter, and told them that I would live a while longer.

HELLINGER What about the father of your child?

GERTRUDE We have been separated for two years. We weren't married. His brother committed suicide a few years ago, and his parents are also divorced.

HELLINGER We'll set up a constellation with three people: you, your child, and the father of your child.

142

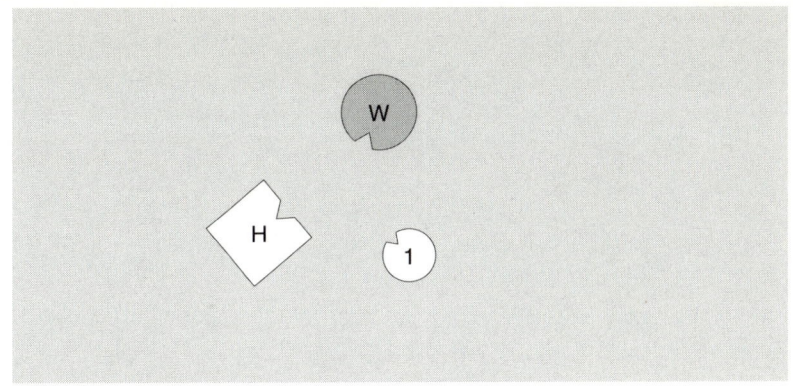

H   Husband
W   Woman (Gertrude)
1   Only Child, a daughter, handicapped – spastic

When Gertrude has finished setting up the representatives, she sits down again, crying.

HELLINGER *after a while* I'll put you in your own place immediately. *As she takes her place* Now, straighten up inside, to your full greatness. Close your eyes and feel all the dead behind you wishing you well. Now, look at your daughter out of this strength and say to her, "Dear child."
GERTRUDE Dear child.
HELLINGER "I take you to me."
GERTRUDE I take you to me.
HELLINGER "I am always your mother."
GERTRUDE I am always your mother.
HELLINGER Take her to you.

Gertrude goes to her daughter and they embrace warmly. Gertrude rocks her gently.

HELLINGER *after a while* Stand next to her and put your arm around her.

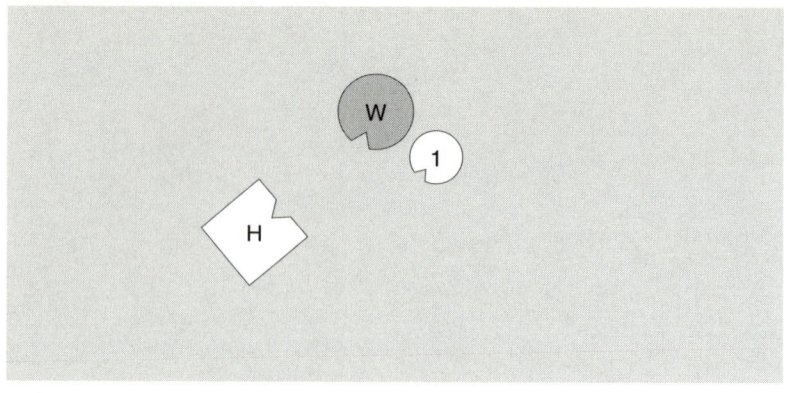

HELLINGER *to Gertrude* How are you feeling?

GERTRUDE A bit freer.

HELLINGER You have to stay large. Look at the father of your child and tell him, "No matter what you do, I remain her mother."

GERTRUDE No matter what you do, I remain her mother.

HELLINGER How is that?

GERTRUDE I feel a bit bigger.

HELLINGER Yes, the appropriate size.

To daughter How are you feeling?

DAUGHTER I feel good next to her. There was a big difference when you said, "Think about the dead behind you." She got bigger then.

HELLINGER *to husband* How about you?

HUSBAND I feel a longing for this woman. The daughter doesn't play much of a role for me.

HELLINGER Stand next to your daughter and put your arm around her.

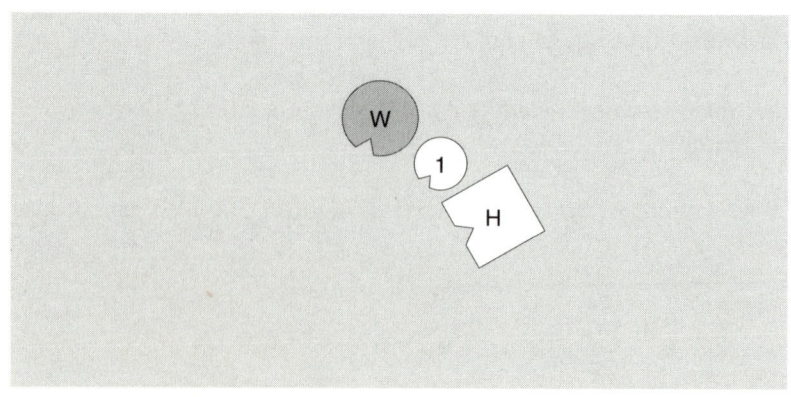

HELLINGER *to husband* How is that?

HUSBAND *hesitating* Strange.

HELLINGER *to daughter* And for you?

DAUGHTER For me it feels good. I was already sensing his strength before and wanting it.

HELLINGER *to Gertrude* And for you?

GERTRUDE The first thing I was aware of was how solid she seems. I think it's nice to have him standing there.

HELLINGER Look at him and say, "Please."

GERTRUDE Please.

HELLINGER *to man* Say, "Yes."

HUSBAND Yes.

HELLINGER How is that?

HUSBAND Good.

HELLINGER *looking at Gertrude* Sometimes miracles happen in the soul. Can we leave it like that?

GERTRUDE *nodding* It's fine.

HELLINGER Okay, that's it.

"I'M DOING FINE"
Husband died in car accident caused by his wife

PARTICIPANT Last year, a couple wanted to attend a course of mine. They were relatives of my wife that we had just recently got to know. Shortly before the seminar, I received the news that they had been in a car accident. The wife was driving and she was at fault. Her husband died in the accident, and she was seriously injured and almost died. She survived, however, and it looks as if she will recover. I'm going to visit her soon, and I'm very nervous about it. I don't know what to say to her.

HELLINGER The woman will want to follow her husband into death. Set up a constellation of the woman and her dead husband.

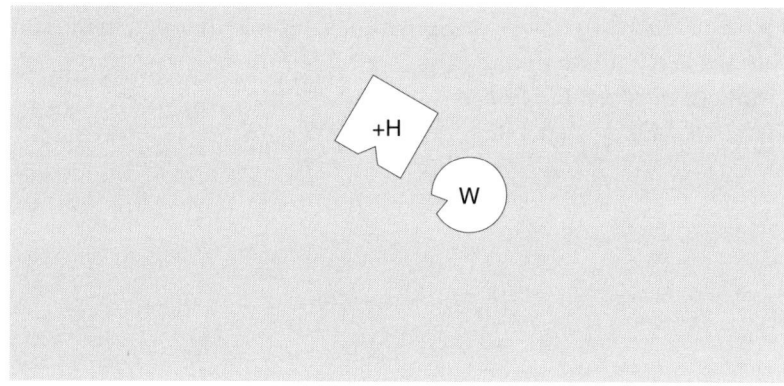

W   Wife
+H   Husband, died in car accident caused by his wife

The man looks at his wife, and she looks straight ahead. Then he looks straight ahead, and she looks at him. After a while, their glances cross briefly. The woman immediately looks straight ahead again, but the man looks at her for a long time. As her eyes move towards him, he turns away and looks straight ahead again. After a while, the man looks over at his wife and then down to the floor. They look directly at each other briefly, but she looks away. The woman breathes deeply, makes a gesture of helplessness with her left hand and begins to cry. The man looks away, then at the floor, then at his wife. They look at each other for a while longer this time before the woman looks away. The man looks at the floor, then at his wife.

HELLINGER How is the husband doing?
HUSBAND I'm doing fine. I'm very much in touch with myself, and I can see clearly. I feel very connected.
HELLINGER Tell her, "I'm doing fine."
HUSBAND I'm doing fine.

The woman looks at her husband briefly, sighs deeply, then looks away.

HELLINGER *to woman* Look at him.
To man Tell her again, "I'm doing fine."
As the woman looks away again You have to look at him.
HUSBAND I'm doing fine.

The woman looks at him and is very moved. She cries and then looks away again.

HELLINGER *to woman* What is it?
WIFE My teeth are chattering and my hands are very heavy.
HELLINGER Look at him.
To man Say it again.
HUSBAND I'm doing fine.
HELLINGER *to woman* Breathe deeply with your mouth open, and look at him – keep looking at him.

She looks at her husband. Hellinger moves her a bit further away.

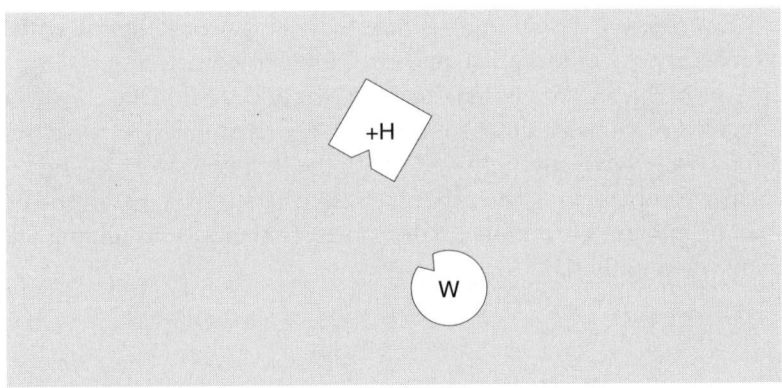

HELLINGER *to husband* How is that for you?

HUSBAND *hesitating* I feel a rejection.
HELLINGER Tell her, "I'm doing fine."
HUSBAND I'm doing fine.
HELLINGER "And I have time."
HUSBAND And I have time. *He smiles at her.*
HELLINGER *to wife* How is that?
WIFE Better.
HELLINGER Tell him, "I'll come, too."
WIFE I'll come, too.
HELLINGER "After a while."
WIFE After a while.
HELLINGER *to husband* How was that?
HUSBAND Nice.
HELLINGER *to wife* And for you?
WIFE Good.

HELLINGER *to participant who raised the issue* Is that okay for you?
PARTICIPANT Yes.
HELLINGER *to representatives* That's good. That was it.

HELLINGER *to group* The process is always the same. The survivors have to allow themselves to be looked at by the dead. That's it. They move into the view of the dead. Then it's impossible for them to follow the dead. To stand before them is more difficult than closing your eyes and dying. There is a magnitude in looking. Isn't it nice that the dead can say, "I'm doing fine"? That's the way it is.

In a course in Hamburg recently, there was a constellation with a woman whose grandfather had shot Jewish women and children. He was in the SS. We put ten dead Jewish children into the constellation. One of them said that for him, death was nothing personal and didn't really have anything to do with the perpetrator. That's how it is, and you have to look at that here, too. There are greater powers than us making life and death decisions. That is very humbling and there is strength in it.

148

ALMA I would like to ask you to help us bring some order into our relationship. I am my husband's third wife and he's my second husband. For me, things don't seem to be in order, and I have the feeling that in our family we aren't in the right place.

HELLINGER What does the husband have to say about it?

GODFREY I'm curious, and I'd be very happy if you could help her.

Laughter in the group

HELLINGER I'll help with one sentence.

To wife Leave him alone.

After a thoughtful pause Just imagine this. There are two heaps of rubble. One belongs to you and one belongs to him. Compare the size of these two piles. How do they compare?

WOMAN I think mine is smaller.

HELLINGER How much smaller?

ALMA Perhaps a third the size of his.

HELLINGER Good estimate. But you act as if …

ALMA … as if they were the same size?

HELLINGER No, as if you were the only one who had one.

ALMA I'm afraid you've got me on that one. I don't understand.

HELLINGER You take over the responsibility for his wreckage. The resolution is for you to leave him to his own pile of rubble.

ALMA Yes, I think so, too.

HELLINGER I'm not going to do anything more.

ALMA Thanks, that's enough.

HELLINGER What's the issue?

BABETTE I had breast cancer twelve years ago and had chemotherapy. A few years later I got ovarian tumors, as well as uterine tumors. Since that time I've suffered from chronic exhaustion which is getting worse.

HELLINGER Are you married?

BABETTE I'm in a relationship. I was married once and divorced, and then my ex-husband died. In a second relationship, the man said he wouldn't marry me and that if I got pregnant he would go back to his homeland. I got pregnant, but I didn't realize it, nor did my doctor. I was in treatment for months because I was in such pain, and after that I felt I had no choice but to abort the child. I couldn't imagine raising a damaged child by myself.

HELLINGER We'll set up you, this man, and the child.

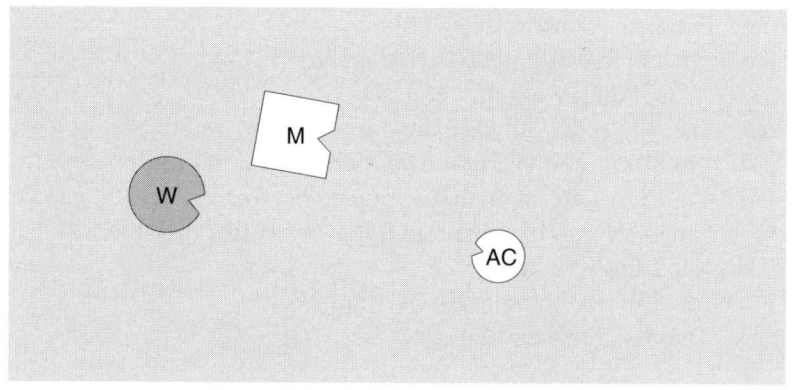

M   Man   AC   Aborted Child
W   Woman (Babette)

HELLINGER *to Babette* How are you?

BABETTE I'm all stirred up.

HELLINGER How is the child doing?

ABORTED CHILD *sighing* My hands are sweaty and my heart is pounding. My legs can hardly hold me up. I'm having trouble standing up.

HELLINGER Sit down.

To man And you?

MAN At first I felt like I wanted to leave, that this had nothing to do with me. Then there was an eerie feeling from behind me. When the child came in I thought she might interest me.

HELLINGER *to Babette's representative* What's going on with you?

WOMAN My heart was pounding incredibly. Now my legs feel very heavy and I'm shaking.

HELLINGER Sit down next to her.

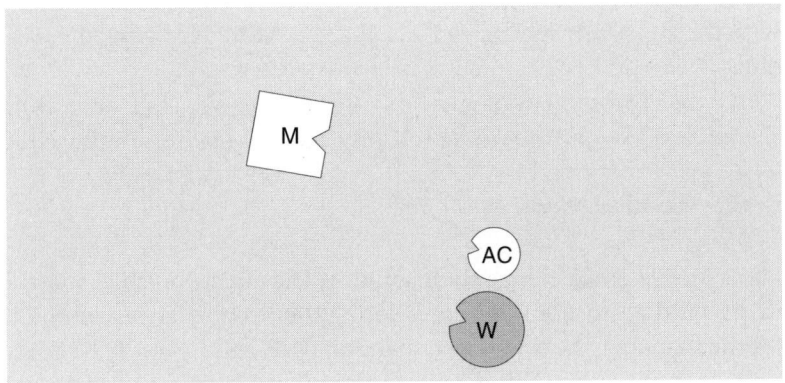

The mother and child keep looking at each other and then looking away. Periodically, they look over at the man.

HELLINGER *after a while, to group* This woman is hardened. She doesn't have any feelings for this dead child.

After a while The man has no feelings for the child either.

After another pause, to aborted child Lie down on your side.

The child lies down on her side with her back to her mother.

HELLINGER *after a pause, to Babette's representative* What's going on with you?

WOMAN I'm so terribly sorry that I can't react to this child. Actually, I like her. But, somehow, I don't have any feelings.

HELLINGER Exactly.

WOMAN It makes me really sad.

HELLINGER That's not a sadness with strength. There's nothing to be done with the mother. You have to remember what she said before,

151

how she justified this, and what the man said. Here, that's all beside the point. There's nothing to be done. Often, illness or death are the only way out. Without love, nothing can happen here. I'll leave this.
HELLINGER *to representative of the aborted child* How was that for you?
ABORTED CHILD *sighing* Miserable, lonely, lost.
HELLINGER *to all representatives* Get yourselves out of these difficult roles.
After a while, to Babette What do you have to say about this?

crying Somehow, it's not complete. Two months ago, I made contact with the child and apologized, because I couldn't see any other way out.
HELLINGER You can't apologize and ask for forgiveness from a child. That doesn't work. That's just self-pity, not real feelings for the child.

Babette is very emotional and crying.

HELLINGER *to group* The only resolution I could see in this situation that would be appropriate, considering the circumstances, would be for the woman to lie down next to the aborted child. Simply lie down, with no hope of anything, just lie down and be there, and be prepared for any consequences. That would have a healing effect in the soul. If you really consider the gravity of this, there is unimaginable pain.
To Babette Sometimes children like this act as angels for their parents.

Babette nods.

HELLINGER Can we leave it like that?

BABETTE Yes.

152

PARTICIPANT Could you say something about a non-resolution, about a situation that goes right to the edge?

HELLINGER The so-called non-resolution is a step within a larger context. I don't know what's going to come out of it, but I take it very seriously that there's no resolution. It's important to recognize the gravity of it.

Illness is sometimes an angel of God. You can see illness as a message from God. But if you don't look, you won't see or hear what's wrong. This is a whole different level of dealing with illness and with fate, where personal plans and wishes don't play any role. If you don't respect the angel, he withdraws. You can see, in this, what kind of an inner transformation is necessary for this kind of work, and also what kind of transformation is made possible.

A therapist who works in this way is a warrior, and must go to the outer limits without fear or blame. Then, everything is regarded with the gravity it really has, and nothing is trivialized. Then things can move on. If you can go straight to the edge, the chances of a resolution are greater than if you turn back and cover things up with nice thoughts and words.

"PLEASE, HOLD ME TIGHT"
Melkersson-Rosenthal syndrome

HELLINGER *to Stella* What is the matter with you?

STELLA I have Melkersson-Rosenthal syndrome.

HELLINGER *to Professor Kaspar Rhyner* Could you explain what that is?

PROFESSOR It's a disease characterized by facial swelling. Sometimes the tongue swells up as well, so that the patient can't speak, or there may be damage to cranial nerves.

HELLINGER So, this is a very serious disease?

PROFESSOR Yes.

HELLINGER *to Stella* How have you managed so far?

STELLA Sometimes better, sometimes worse. It hasn't been easy.

HELLINGER We'll set up two people, you and your illness. Choose two representatives and place them where it feels right to you.

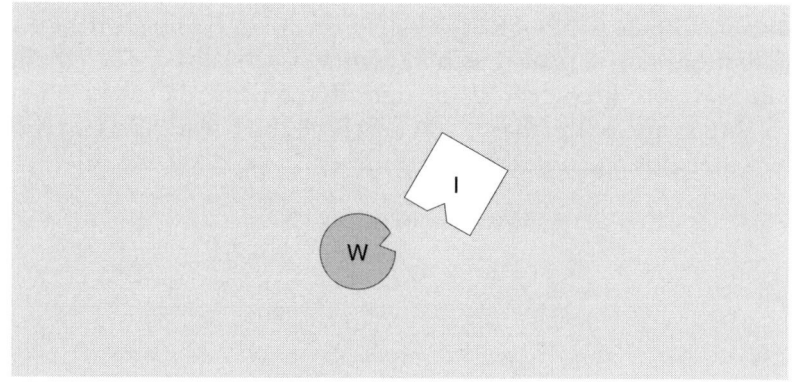

| W | Woman (Stella) | I | Illness |

HELLINGER *to the representatives* Both of you stay very collected and pay attention to whatever movement comes from within. Follow those movements without saying anything.

The woman keeps looking at the representative of the illness. The illness representative moves his arms helplessly about, but remains where he is. Then he reaches out his right hand towards the woman. She moves off to the side and slowly moves around to the right until she is behind him.

154

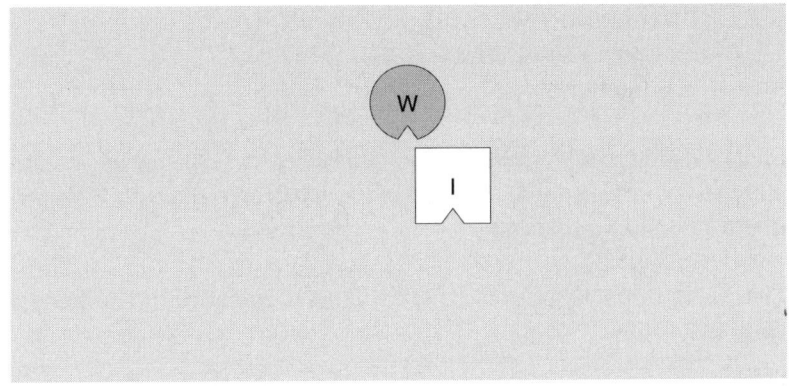

After a while he looks around at her, steps to the side to look over at her, and then steps back. The woman leans against his back. She then sinks to her knees, with her arms around his legs.

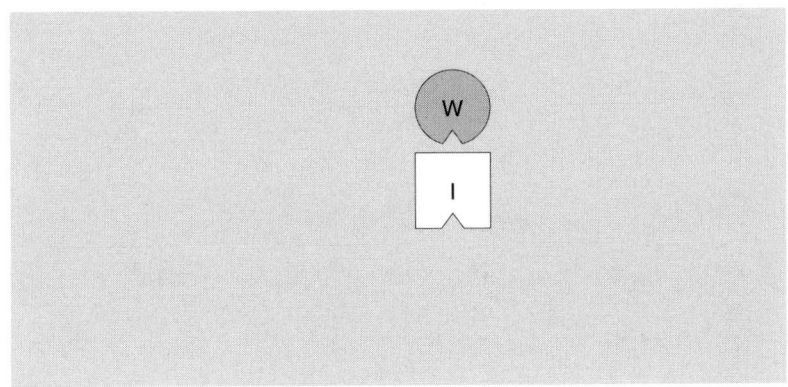

Stella begins to sob and leans against Hellinger. He puts his arm around her. She sobs as if in pain.

HELLINGER Breathe quietly, without making a sound. Calmly, with your mouth open.

Stella quiets down and breathes deeply. The representative of the illness looks down at Stella's representative. He bends down towards her and reaches out his right hand to her. As she raises her head slowly, he touches her gently.

HELLINGER *to Stella* Say, "I'll come, too."

155

STELLA I'll come, too. *She breathes deeply and sighs.*
HELLINGER *after a pause* How was that for you?
STELLA A bit better.

Stella's representative straightens up somewhat, but remains on her knees and puts her arms around the knees of the other representative. He continues to look back around at her.

HELLINGER *to the representative of the illness* Turn around to her and raise her up.

The representative pulls Stella's representative up to him and puts his arm around her. She lays her head on his chest and cries. He puts his hand gently on her head.

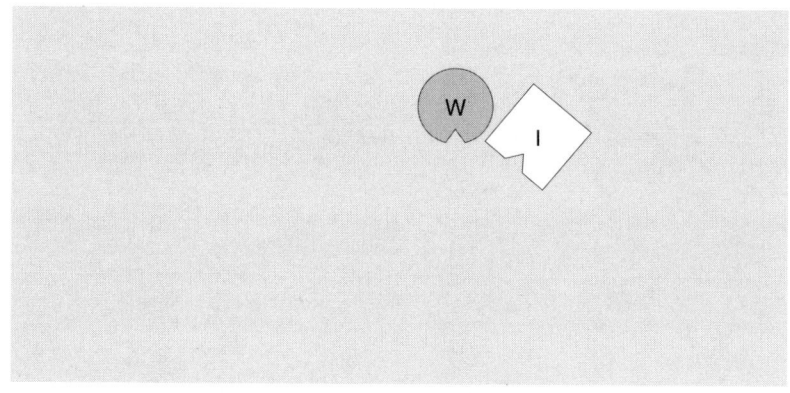

Stella, leaning against Hellinger, sobbing loudly.

HELLINGER Breathe deeply with your mouth open. Without any sound. Breathe deeply.
After a while Who did you lose when you were a child? Who did you lose?
STELLA When I was a child?
HELLINGER Who died?
STELLA My mother died very young and also my father.

Stella's representative loosens her embrace, but the two representatives remain in contact.

HELLINGER *to Stella's representative* How are you feeling?
WOMAN Lighter, but my muscles are like cotton wool.
HELLINGER *to the representative of the illness* And you?
ILLNESS I feel better now. At the beginning, I felt really shaky, and I alternated between waves of heat and cold.
HELLINGER Tell her, "I'll hold you tight."
ILLNESS I'll hold you tight.
HELLINGER Do it. Hold her very tightly.

The two representatives embrace warmly. Stella breathes deeply and sobs. Hellinger puts his arm around her again.

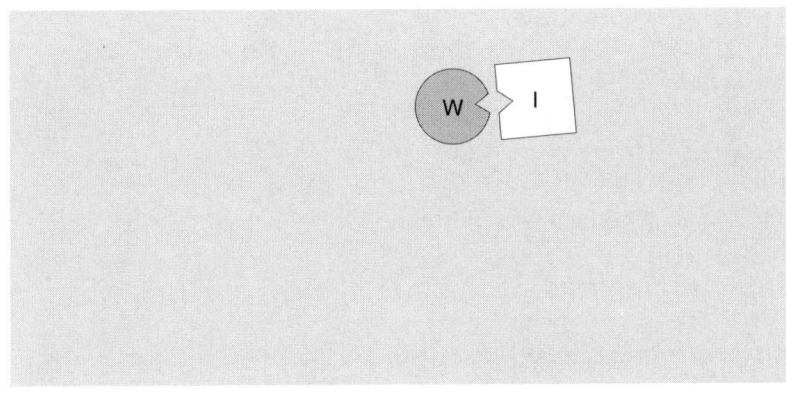

HELLINGER *to Stella* Open your eyes and let yourself be held by your mother and your father. Open your eyes. Look into their faces and say, "Please, hold me tight."
STELLA Please, hold me tight.

Stella closes her eyes and is very still.

HELLINGER *after a while* How are you feeling now?
STELLA I feel better.
HELLINGER Let that work quietly in your soul. Don't talk about it with anyone. Don't let anyone persuade you to do that. Just keep it in your soul and your soul will help you. Okay?
STELLA Yes. Thank you.
HELLINGER Gladly done.
To the representatives You were very sensitive and you've performed a great service. Thank you very much.

157

HELLINGER *after a while, to Stella* We have a great friend you know. Each of us has a very special, great friend. You certainly have one. Perhaps you've never thought about it as having a great friend.
STELLA No, I don't know him.
HELLINGER People used to call him, Friend Hein. You probably don't know that expression here in Switzerland. Friend Hein?
STELLA I don't know him.
HELLINGER That's death.

Stella nods.

HELLINGER He is the greatest.
STELLA Yes.
HELLINGER And he's very calm.
STELLA Yes.
HELLINGER Very still.
STELLA Yes.
HELLINGER You can depend on him.
STELLA Yes.
HELLINGER If you have him at your side.
STELLA Yes.

Hellinger and Stella look at each other calmly and companionably.

HELLINGER I'll tell you a story about this friend.

Somewhere, far far away, where once the Wild West lay, a man with a rucksack on his back walked through a vast land, devoid of people. After hours of walking the sun was high in the sky and his thirst was great. He saw a farmhouse on the horizon and thought, "Thank God! Finally, another human being in all this loneliness. I'll stop there and ask for something to drink. Perhaps we'll sit on the veranda and talk for a while before I go on." And he imagined how pleasant that would be.

As he came closer to the farmhouse, however, he could see that the farmer was working in the garden, and he began to have doubts. "Perhaps he has a lot to do, and if I tell him what I want, he'll be inconvenienced and he won't like me interrupting him." As he approached the garden gate, he waved at the farmer and walked on past.

From the farmer's point of view, as he saw the traveler in the distance, he was overjoyed. "Thank God! Finally, another human being in all this loneliness. Hopefully he'll stop in. We could have a drink of something together and perhaps we'll sit on the veranda and talk a while before he goes on." And he went into the house to prepare something to drink.

As the stranger drew nearer, however, the farmer began to have doubts. "He's most probably in a hurry and if I tell him what I want, he'll feel inconvenienced and might think I'm being very demanding. But, perhaps he's thirsty and will stop of his own accord. The best thing to do is to go into the front garden and act as if I'm very busy. Then, he'll see me and if he wants to stop, he'll say something." As the stranger waved and walked on by, he said, "What a pity."

The stranger walked on and the sun got higher in the sky and his thirst grew greater. It was hours before he saw another farmhouse. He said to himself, "This time I'm going to stop whether it's inconvenient or not. I'm so thirsty, I have to have something to drink."

This farmer saw the stranger from afar and thought, "I hope he doesn't stop here. I have too much to do, and can't always be taking care of other people." He went on with his work without looking up.

The stranger saw him in the field and went to him and said, "I'm very thirsty. Please, could you give me something to drink?" The farmer thought, "I can't just send him away, after all, he's a human being too." He led the stranger into the house and brought him something to drink.

159

The stranger said, "I was looking at your garden. It's easy to see that there's an expert at work here, who loves plants and knows what they need." The farmer was very pleased and said, "I see you know something about it." And they sat down and talked for a long time.

Then, the stranger stood and said, "It's time for me to move on." The farmer protested. "Look," he said, "the sun is already low. Why don't you stay the night here? We could sit on the veranda a while and talk, and you could go on your way tomorrow." The stranger agreed to stay.

That evening they sat on the veranda, and the vast land lay transfigured by the dusk. As darkness came, the stranger began to tell a story about his life and how his world had changed ever since the moment he had become aware that in every step he took he was accompanied by someone. At first he hadn't believed that there was someone going everywhere with him. He couldn't believe that when he stood still, the other stood still, and when he started off again, the other did as well. It took a long time before he understood who this companion was.

"My constant companion," he said, "is my death. I've got so used to him now that I would miss him if he weren't there. He is my truest and best friend. When I don't know the right thing to do or how to proceed, I remain quiet for a moment and wait for his answer. I put myself completely at his mercy and I know that he is there and I am here. And without taking any notice of my own thoughts, I wait for a signal to come from him. If I remain collected and courageous, a word comes from him to me like a flash of lightning lighting up the sky – and I feel clear."

The farmer found this talk very strange and gazed silently into the night. After a long time, he too saw his own companion, his own death, and bowed down before him. It seemed to him that the rest of his life was transformed into something as precious as love in the awareness of parting, and as filled to overflowing as love.

The next morning they had breakfast together and the farmer said, "Even though you're leaving, a friend remains with me." They walked outside and shook hands. The stranger continued on his way and the farmer returned to his field.

HELLINGER *to Stella* So, now I've told you a long story. Okay, that's all. All the best to you.

STELLA Thank you very much.

VERENA I suffer from a manic-depressive illness, and I also have psoriasis.

HELLINGER Manics fly away.

VERENA Thank God, I haven't yet experienced a true manic state. My doctor says that I have sub-manic states.

HELLINGER I see. But the others will come.

VERENA I hope not.

HELLINGER Well, if the doctor says "not yet", then they're sure to come later.

VERENA I live with that fear chasing me. *She begins to cry.*

HELLINGER Yes, of course. That's what happens with diagnoses. *Verena sighs deeply.* That's the effect. You can make up a parcel to send to your psychiatrist. Inside the parcel, you put a tiny packet, labeled "sub-mania" and send it back to him with best wishes.

VERENA I don't understand.

HELLINGER Shall I start again, from the beginning?

VERENA I didn't understand.

HELLINGER Okay. The psychiatrist has given you a double-edged gift. He pushed something off on you, namely, a sub-mania. So, you can pack it up again and send it back to him with best wishes.

VERENA Oh, I just got it. He told me that every time I'm feeling good, It's probably a "sub-mania". *Loud laughter in the group.*

HELLINGER If someone is really feeling high, then it's a sub-mania. Have you ever seen someone really rejoicing?

VERENA Yes, often.

HELLINGER They're all manic. There's no other way to explain someone rejoicing, sometimes even jumping into the air. You'd have to think they're all in a manic state. I'd say, change therapists, or better yet, do without one for a while.

VERENA My depressions come often and they're increasing.

HELLINGER Depression – that's something else again. Do you know what depression means?

VERENA *furiously* I think, rage and aggression. *She weeps.*

HELLINGER Well, that's another assumption. No. But, all of a sudden you had a lot of energy. It suits you. *She laughs.* Someone feels depressive when they're missing their mother or father. Is that so with you?

VERENA Yes, my father died very young.

HELLINGER Yes, that's it. You see? That's it. If you take him into your heart, you'll feel joyful, but the normal sort. *She laughs.* Okay, we'll set up a constellation with you and your father.

Verena places the representatives next to one another. They spontaneously put an arm around each other.

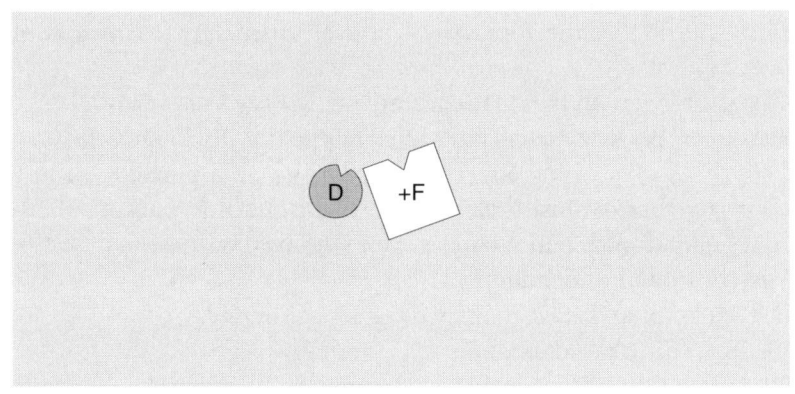

+F   Father, who died young
D   Daughter (Verena)

HELLINGER *to the representatives* Follow your impulses, whatever seems right.

Father and daughter put their heads together, tenderly.

HELLINGER *to Verena* You see, that's it. There's the resolution of depression. How old were you when your father died?

VERENA I was one year and two and a half months.

HELLINGER That's much too young. Such a young child can't mourn. Did you know that? The child feels angry instead of mourning, sometimes. But, that anger is only love, pure love. Look at that.

162

The two representatives touch each other gently, as if with deep grief. He puts his hand on her head, and she holds his arm.

As Verena watches this, she sobs loudly and leans against Hellinger. He puts his arm around her.

HELLINGER *to Verena* You see, that's it. It's something very simple, and very human. It can be understood at a deep level.
After a while, as Verena calms down Look at that picture. A child needs a father. That's the true secret of your depression.

The representative of the father strokes the head and shoulder of his daughter, very gently. Verena sits up and her crying stops for a while, then begins again. Hellinger puts his arm around her once more.

HELLINGER Who is really sad?
VERENA *crying* My father is sad.
HELLINGER Yes, he is sad.
VERENA Yes.
HELLINGER Tell him, "I'll carry it with you."
VERENA Papa, I'll carry it with you. *She cries:* I think he was often sad.
HELLINGER When a father dies so young and knows that his child is left behind, he is sad. Now, look at him again and tell him, "You should get some pleasure from me."
VERENA Father, you should get some pleasure from me. Yes. *She sobs.*
HELLINGER Tell him, "I've grown up."
VERENA I've grown up.
HELLINGER "You should get some pleasure from me."
VERENA You should … *she breathes deeply and sighs.*
HELLINGER Open your eyes and look at him. Say it in a normal voice. "Papa, you should get some pleasure from me."
VERENA *still sobbing* Father, you should get some pleasure from me.
HELLINGER Say it in a completely normal voice.
VERENA *in a calm voice* Father, you should get some pleasure from me.
HELLINGER "And I hold a place for you in my heart."
VERENA And I hold … *she sobs.*
HELLINGER You have to look at him.
VERENA *sobbing* And I hold a place for you in my heart.

163

HELLINGER Tell him, "In my heart, you can even be joyful."

VERENA *calmly* In my heart, you can even be joyful.

HELLINGER *indicating the representative of the father* He's lighting up. Can you see how his face has lit up?

To father's representative How are you doing?

FATHER I'm smiling.

HELLINGER Okay, we'll leave it there. That was it.

To Verena Okay?

VERENA Yes.

I'LL LIE WITH YOU
Chronic pain syndrome

HELLINGER *to Ludwig* What is your issue?

LUDWIG I have been very ill for the past two years. Now I've developed a chronic pain syndrome that won't let up, and I can't get any sleep. I gave up, or lost, my job. I was burned out, completely exhausted. Every time I thought I'd reached the bottom, things got worse.

HELLINGER Close your eyes.

After a while Hellinger bows Ludwig's head slightly and places his hand on Ludwig's back, between the shoulder blades.

HELLINGER Keep your eyes closed, and open your mouth slightly. Bow your head a bit more. That's it.

After a while And now let yourself sink down to the bottom … keep breathing … all the way down to the bottom.

Ludwig is crying.

HELLINGER Give in. Just give in … and now, lie down next to someone … next to someone … at the bottom … absolutely still.

Ludwig leans forward in a deeper bow.

HELLINGER Give in. Let go.

Tears roll down Ludwig's face. After a while he sighs deeply.

HELLINGER Inside yourself, say, "Here's where I stay."

Ludwig becomes quieter.

HELLINGER That's right. "Here's where I stay."

After a while Go where it's still, and stay there.

After a while Hellinger removes his hand from Ludwig's back. After another pause, Ludwig sighs deeply, and then breathes more easily. After a few more minutes he leans back, exhales and looks at Hellinger.

HELLINGER I'll leave it there. Is that okay?

Ludwig nods.

The following day

HELLINGER *to Ludwig* How are you doing with your pains?
LUDWIG Better, yes. They're still there, but less so.
HELLINGER That's nice. Are you married?
LUDWIG Yes.
HELLINGER Have you got any children?
LUDWIG Two – no, three. One child is from my first marriage.
HELLINGER How old are your children?
LUDWIG My daughter from the first marriage is sixteen, and the two boys from my second marriage are six and eight.
HELLINGER Why did your first marriage break up?
LUDWIG I don't know. My first wife just said at some point that it was over for her.
HELLINGER We'll set up a constellation of your present system. That is, your first wife, your daughter, your second wife, and your two sons.

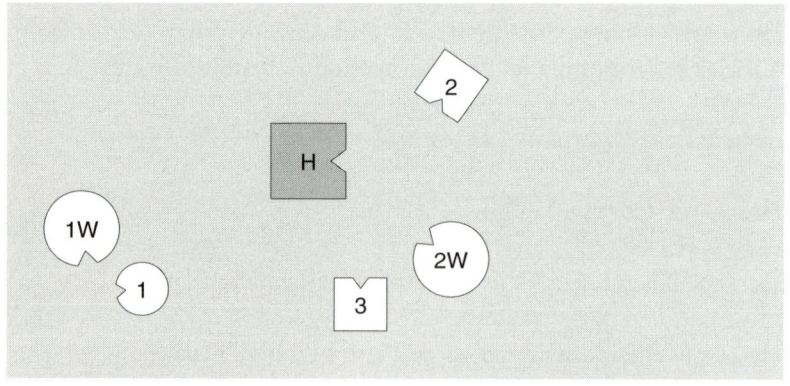

H	Husband (Ludwig)	1	First Child, a daughter
1W	First Wife	2W	Second Wife
		2	Second Child, a son
		3	Third Child, a son

Hellinger *indicating Ludwig's representative* He wants to leave.

Ludwig I don't know what that means.

Hellinger He wants to die.

Ludwig Yes. But not just that.

Hellinger Hopefully. He's being drawn somewhere. Where is the pull?

Ludwig Towards my home, where I came from.

Hellinger What happened in your family of origin?

Ludwig What seemed really meaningful here yesterday, is that my grandfather died when I was 16 months old.

Hellinger What did he die of?

Ludwig Stomach cancer.

Hellinger No, that can't be it. Did anything else happen?

Ludwig Another death that didn't seem important up until now, was my great-grandmother, the mother of my grandmother, who was a very important person for me. This great-grandmother died giving birth.

Hellinger Add a representative for this great-grandmother.

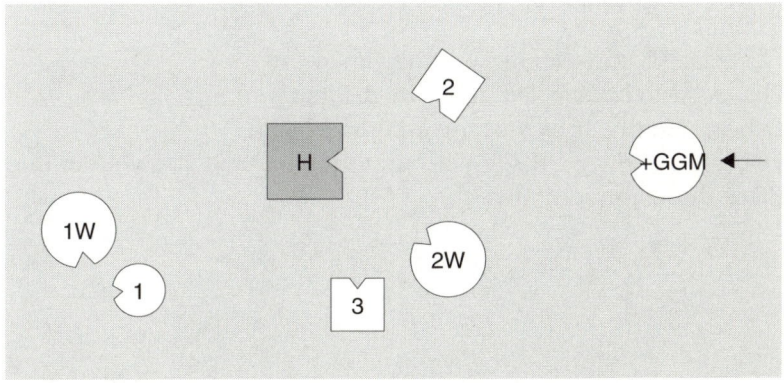

+GGM   Great-grandmother (mother's mother's mother,
        who died giving birth)

Hellinger *to Ludwig's representative* What's the matter?

Husband At first I felt some kind of accusation from my second wife. Now that the great-grandmother is here, I feel guilty. I want to turn away. I can't stand it.

Hellinger Go and stand next to her.

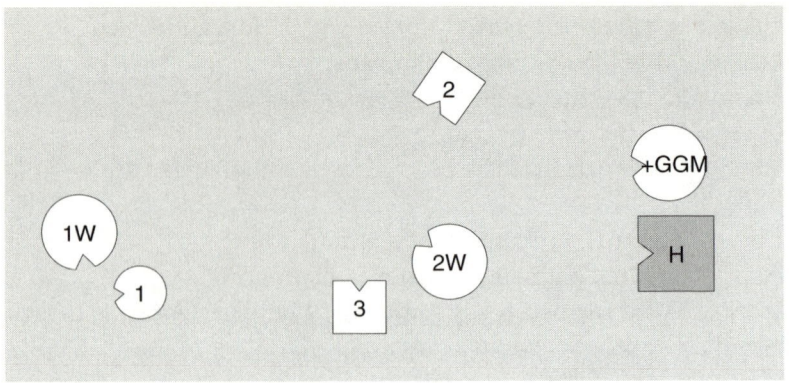

HELLINGER The great-grandmother has to take him in her arms and hold him tight.

The great-grandmother's representative puts her arms around Ludwig's representative. He sobs loudly. After a while, he releases her embrace and looks at her. Both representatives are radiant.

HELLINGER How quickly that happens. How's the great-grandmother feeling?
GREAT GRANDMOTHER I feel overwhelmed.
HELLINGER *to Ludwig* Did the baby die, too?
LUDWIG No, the baby was my grandmother.
HELLINGER Now we'll add your grandmother and also your mother. Place those representatives.

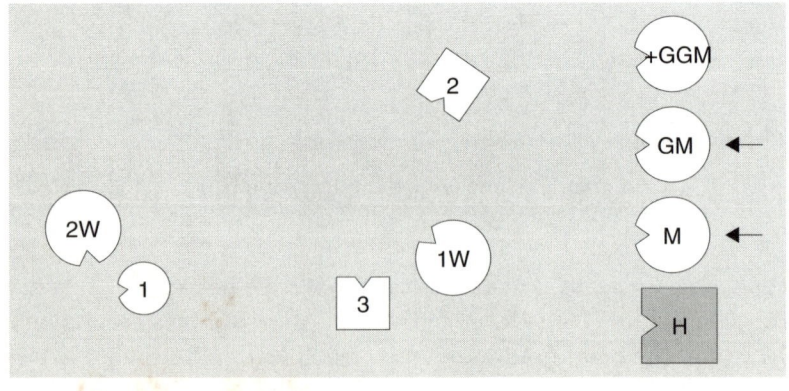

GM Grandmother (mother's mother)   M   Mother

HELLINGER *to Ludwig's representative* How do you feel, now?

HUSBAND Much calmer. I know now that I'm her great-grandson. I'm not guilty.

HELLINGER How is the first wife feeling?

FIRST WIFE I have mixed feelings. I feel like he's to blame that I don't really have contact with my daughter. I sense her reproach that I left, but I feel like I didn't have any choice except to leave. When you said that he wanted to die, my spontaneous thought was, "Right. It'd serve him right." I shocked myself thinking that and had to really look at him. When the great-grandmother came in, I felt relieved and thought, "Finally!" The thing with my daughter bothers me a lot. I would like to have a good relationship with her, but I can't reach her.

HELLINGER *to daughter* And for you?

FIRST CHILD I feel really pressured by my mother. There are so many demands. I feel like I'm the mother. I'm completely cut off from all the others. That doesn't have anything to do with me.

HELLINGER *to representatives* Okay, come with me.

Hellinger places the representatives in the natural order.

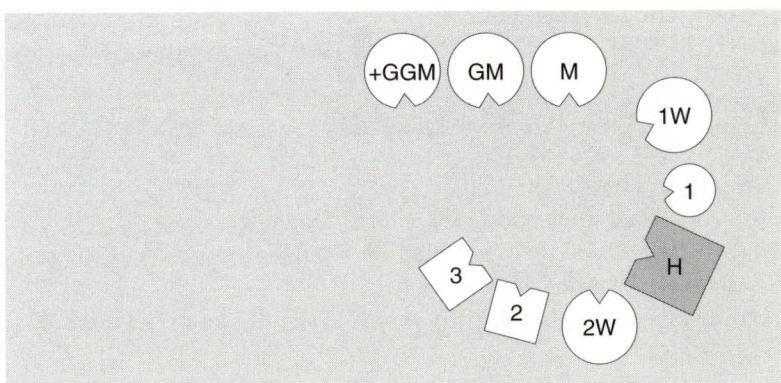

HELLINGER *to daughter* How is it now?

FIRST CHILD Better.

FIRST WIFE It's easier, but there's still some pressure.

HUSBAND *to first wife* I have the feeling that I've never seen you before this. Now I see someone there. *They nod to each other.* I'm sorry.

HELLINGER There was an entanglement with the fate of your great-grandmother. Because of that, you couldn't see your first wife.

To second wife How are you feeling here?

SECOND WIFE It's better. I felt overwhelmed. I couldn't make any contact with my eldest son, and I kept wanting to say that I just couldn't do everything alone, and that I couldn't reach my children. Now it's better.

In the meantime, the daughter and mother have been smiling at each other and they put an arm around each other.

SECOND CHILD Now I feel embedded in this family. Before I didn't.

THIRD CHILD I have the same feeling. Before I felt so much pressure from the left side, from the first wife and her daughter. I had no relationship with my mother. Now it's better.

Ludwig takes his own place in the constellation and looks around at all the representatives.

HELLINGER *to Ludwig* Tell your first wife too, "Now, I see you."

LUDWIG Now I see you.

HELLINGER "And I respect you."

LUDWIG And I respect you.

HELLINGER Tell your daughter, "Now I see your mother."

LUDWIG Now I see your mother.

HELLINGER "And I respect her."

LUDWIG And I respect her.

FIRST CHILD Thank you.

FIRST WIFE That feels good. *She smiles at Ludwig.*

HELLINGER *to second wife* Tell his first wife, "I honor you as the first."

SECOND WIFE I honor you as the first.

HELLINGER "Please be friendly when I take this man now, and keep him."

SECOND WIFE Please be friendly when I take this man now, and keep him.

FIRST WIFE Yes. *She nods at the second wife.*

HELLINGER *to Ludwig* How's that for you?

LUDWIG It turns everything upside down.

HELLINGER And?

LUDWIG *laughs* It's good.

HELLINGER Okay.

To second wife How are you feeling now that you've said that?

170

SECOND WIFE Good. A weight dropped off, and I feel freer.

HELLINGER I think we've got it.

To Ludwig Tell each of your children, "I am your father and I remain your father."

LUDWIG *to each child in turn* I am your father and I remain your father.

HELLINGER Tell your second wife, "I am your husband and I remain your husband."

LUDWIG I am your husband and I remain your husband. *They smile at each other.*

HELLINGER Okay, that was it.

To group The death of a woman giving birth is one of the most momentous events possible in a family. When there is a particularly difficult fate like that, the problem is that people become afraid. There is a feeling that thinking about this fate, or honoring the person who suffered, will make this fate continue on in some way. So, often, it is excluded and feared.

Also, people are often afraid of the dead, afraid that they might be antagonistic or envious. The tombstone on the grave is actually an attempt to keep the dead in the grave so they can't come out. They used to be placed flat on top of the grave to hold the dead in place. There's a very deep fear there. But in this denial and avoidance, what is achieved is exactly what was feared, and the blessings that could come from the dead are excluded.

Here, we go round the other way, and bring the dead into view and honor them. You can see how friendly they are when they're honored.

A previous partner is also often excluded, out of fear that this person might have a negative influence on the new family. In this case, too, the result is negative. Not because the person is bad, but because he or she is not respected and honored. The system won't tolerate someone being excluded or not honored when that person has a right to their place in the system. If you acknowledge this, and for example, have a man say to his former wife, "I've never really seen you." then he can look at her and she will appear friendly. Deep down, people are really friendly when they are respected. Then, the second partnership has more of a depth and a better chance of fulfillment. That's the secret of our work here. It's plain, loving, and human.

HELLINGER *to Trudy, who always appears to be very cheerful and happy*
Shall I work with you now?
TRUDY I'll trust your judgement on that.
HELLINGER How should I know, with your cheerfulness? Come here.

She sits down next to him.

HELLINGER Do you know where people are really cheerful? Someone asked me what Buddha did in Nirvana. The only thing I could imagine is: He laughs.

Trudy laughs.

HELLINGER Your eyes contradict your mouth. Close your eyes.

She closes her eyes and becomes serious and sad. She sighs.

HELLINGER Yes. Breathe deeply. That's it.

Hellinger lays his hand on her back, between the shoulder blades.

HELLINGER Bow forward slightly.
After a while And now cry over your illness. Breathe deeply. Cry over your illness. Bow your head a little bit more.

Trudy is crying and breathing deeply.

HELLINGER Turn yourself over to your pain.
After a while Now, lean on me here.

Trudy rests her head on Hellinger's shoulder and sobs. After a while she straightens up and looks at him.

HELLINGER There's a deep pain in there. You have a very deep pain. Close your eyes again, but stay turned towards me. Where does the child want to lean?

172

TRUDY On my whole family.
HELLINGER On anyone in particular?
TRUDY On my dead brother.

She puts her head back on Hellinger's shoulder and cries.

HELLINGER *after a while* Tell him, "A while longer, then I'll come, too."
TRUDY A while longer, then I'll come, too.
HELLINGER *after a pause* How is that for you?
TRUDY Good.
HELLINGER Yes. For whom do you have to be so happy? Who can't stand the pain?
TRUDY My son.
HELLINGER Oh, yes.

She begins to cry again.

HELLINGER Imagine him standing here in front of you. Tell him, "I'll stay as long as I can."
TRUDY I'll stay as long as I can.
HELLINGER How old is he?
TRUDY Thirty-three.
HELLINGER Tell him, "I'm going my own way."
TRUDY I'm going my own way.
HELLINGER "I'll stay as long as I can, but I'm going my own way."
TRUDY I'll stay as long as I can, but I'm going my own way.

She closes her eyes as she speaks.

HELLINGER Say it in all seriousness. You can't spare him the grief and the pain. That's not yours to do. You have to trust him to handle the grief and the pain himself. Tell him again.
TRUDY I'll stay a while longer if I can, but I'm going my own way. I have to trust that you can handle the grief and the pain.
HELLINGER "I can trust you to do that." Say it like that.
TRUDY I can trust you to do that.
HELLINGER That's it. That had strength. It's also better for him like this. Should I leave it there?
TRUDY Yes.
HELLINGER Okay. That's good.

HELLINGER What is the difficulty?
MELISSA I make my life a living Hell. I am destroying myself.
HELLINGER I'm afraid I don't understand. You have to say it very clearly for me.
MELISSA I'm afraid to get up every morning. I plunge from one crisis to another in a self-destructive pattern.
HELLINGER Who told you that?
MELISSA I feel it myself.
HELLINGER Sometimes people run themselves down when they face God, in the hope that he will look more kindly on them. *Melissa nods.* There are also therapists who are more receptive when clients present themselves badly. I don't regard that in such a positive way.
MELISSA I'm aware of that.
HELLINGER So, very concretely, what is it?
MELISSA For the past five years, I've been scratching my skin to an extreme degree. For about two months now, it's been a constant thing, every day, all day.
HELLINGER That's information enough to work with. That's concrete. How old are you?
MELISSA Twenty-six.
HELLINGER Are you married?
MELISSA No.
HELLINGER Have you got any children?
MELISSA No.
HELLINGER What happened in your family of origin?
MELISSA I've got two older brothers. I know from my mother that she wasn't allowed to have her first child. It was with her first partner, an Englishman, but they killed it. I know that. She came back from England and wasn't allowed to have the child. It was too shameful for the family.
HELLINGER They were pious, of course. The pious do things like that. They kill a child to avoid shame. Terrible. *Melissa nods.* Sinners just accept the child. Was it a boy or a girl?
MELISSA A girl.

174

HELLINGER How far along was the pregnancy?

MELISSA It was in the fifth month. My mother had the baby and my grandmother and my aunt took it and burned it up in the stove.

HELLINGER Was the child aborted?

MELISSA It was aborted, but lived for a while, and then was burned up in the stove.

Hellinger chooses a representative for the dead child and has her lie on her back on the floor. Then he has Melissa lie on her back next to the child.

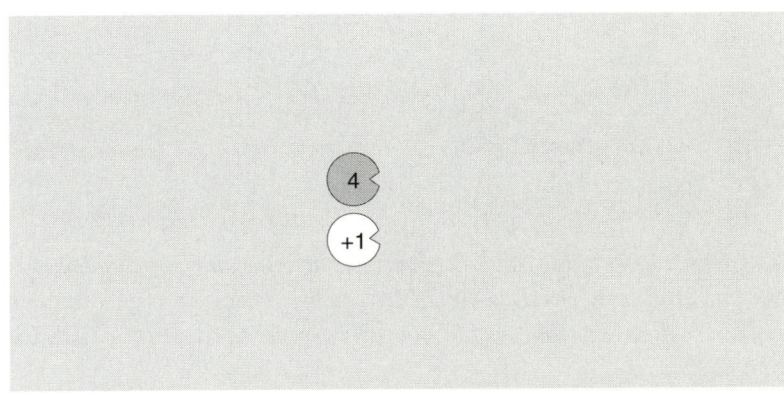

+1   First Child, a daughter, aborted in the fifth month, lived briefly, and was burned in the stove.

4   **Fourth Child, a daughter (Melissa)**

HELLINGER *to representative of the dead child* Close your eyes and lie very still.

To Melissa And look over at her.

Both lie quietly for a while. Then, the dead child looks at her sister. They take hands. Melissa is breathing heavily. After a while, the dead child turns her head away and closes her eyes.

HELLINGER *after a while, to Melissa* Follow any movements you feel.

Melissa lets go of her dead sister's hand, who then looks over at her. They look at each other, then Melissa turns on her side and turns her back to her sister. The dead sister reaches out and strokes Melissa's back and head. Me-

175

lissa breathes heavily. After a while, Hellinger has Melissa stand up and brings her back to her chair. He chooses a representative for the child's mother and places her on her back next to the dead child.

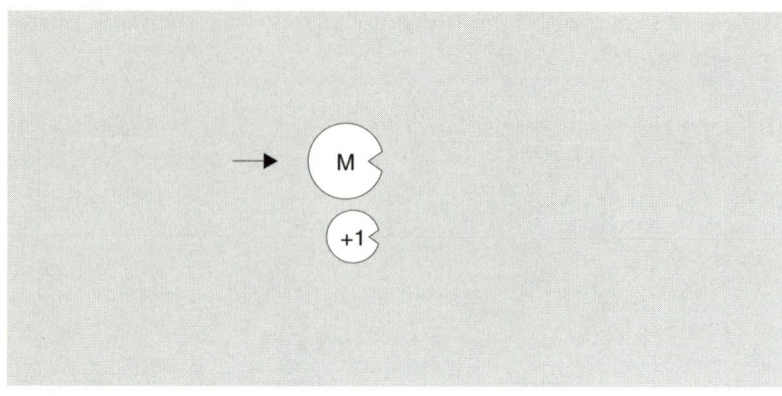

M   Mother

The mother looks at the child, then turns to her. She pulls the child's head to her and strokes it. The dead child turns to her. They embrace warmly and remain so for a long time, as the mother continues to stroke the child's back and head.

HELLINGER *after a while, to Melissa* Do you know what the solution is for you?
MELISSA *breathes heavily and pauses* I have to leave her with my mother.
HELLINGER That's exactly it. Say to her, "Dear Sister,"
MELISSA Dear Sister.
HELLINGER "I leave you with your mother."
MELISSA I leave you with your mother.
HELLINGER Tell your mother, too. What did you call your mother?
MELISSA Mummy.
HELLINGER "Mummy, I leave her with you."
MELISSA Mummy, I leave her with you.
HELLINGER "I'm going to my father now."
MELISSA I'm going to my father, now.
HELLINGER *after a while* You have to let your mother go. And you have to let her die.
MELISSA *breathing deeply and nodding* Yes.

176

HELLINGER Now you move away and go to your father. Being with your father is a good place for you. Agreed?

Melissa nods.

HELLINGER Okay.

Hellinger has the two representatives stand up.

HELLINGER *to the mother's representative* How was that for you?
MOTHER *sighs* There was an incredible sadness and pain.
HELLINGER There's nothing more to hold the mother back.
To the representative of the dead child And for you?
FIRST CHILD When my sister was lying next to me, I was hot down the right side. I wanted to touch her, I wanted to touch her skin, too – but I also wanted to push her away. It was easier for me when she stood up. It was just right when my mother was next to me.
HELLINGER Okay, thank you.

To group Often, when psychotherapists are confronted with such a situation, they often respond to "the poor mother," but there's no saving this mother. There's nothing to do but to die. Does a person want to live after something like that? It's hard to imagine. They have to die. It's the only possible place to find peace.

HELLINGER *to group* During the break, someone spoke to me about an issue. Could I ask that doctor to come up please?
To Laurence Is it okay to work with this now?
LAURENCE Yes.
HELLINGER *to group* I'll tell you the situation. He is a psychiatrist and was attacked by a patient and seriously injured. The patient was trying to kill him.
To Laurence Is that correct?
LAURENCE Yes.
HELLINGER I'd like to set up the constellation of this situation and look at the dynamics, to give you an orientation. We'll take two representatives: you and the patient.

Laurence chooses two representatives and places them.

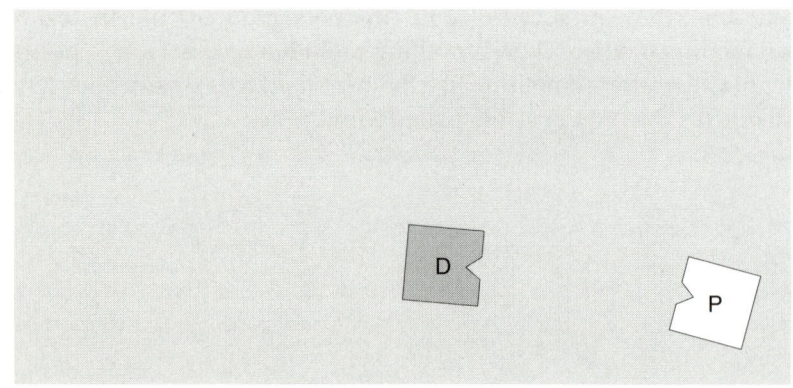

D **Doctor (Laurence)**
P   Patient

They look at each other for a long time. The doctor moves a step towards the patient, but then, after a moment, he steps back again. They continue looking at each other the whole time. After a while, Hellinger leads the doctor away and turns him around.

178

HELLINGER *to Laurence's representative* How is that now?

DOCTOR I'm not as afraid.

HELLINGER *to patient's representative* How is that for you?

PATIENT It's better now that he's gone away.

HELLINGER Yes, exactly.

PATIENT There's no solution. I couldn't resolve it.

HELLINGER *to the representative* Stay where you are for a moment, both of you.

To group I'll explain something. We talked about this earlier and he told me that he had gone back to the patient later to try to resolve the issue. I told him that he couldn't do that. Even a schizophrenic has to stand by the consequences of his actions. If he is dangerous to other people and has to be kept in protective custody. You can't try to free him from that.

To Laurence That way, he has his self-respect. The representative of the patient made it clear that he couldn't do anything. He is incapable. After this act, there's nothing more to be done. You have to leave him to his fate and turn away from him, as we did in the constellation. Does that make sense?

LAURENCE Yes. I feel a mixture of sadness and pain.

HELLINGER That's not your place. You can't be sad about it, nor can you feel pain over him. All that takes away his dignity, and will make him angrier than he is.

Laurence nods.

HELLINGER You have to go all the way to the extreme limit. Is that clear to you?

179

LAURENCE Yes.

HELLINGER Have we saved you?

Laurence laughs.

HELLINGER I mean it seriously. Otherwise, you will be in danger again. A warrior fights.

Laurence nods.

HELLINGER Okay, that's all.
To the representatives Get out of these roles.
To Laurence Is that okay like that?
LAURENCE Yes.

HELLINGER *to group* Are there any questions about this?
PARTICIPANT I'd like to ask a very specific question about what you're saying. I'm also a psychiatrist and have been for forty years. I'm having some trouble with this interpretation. In a situation like that, what I feel is pity, sympathy, and love. My opinion is that a person who is ill is an altered person and out of control.
HELLINGER Yes, that's the other side. The question is, what happens to him if I behave as you suggest, and what happens if I behave as in the constellation? And, what happens in the patient's family, for example if he should have children, if I respond in the one way or in the other? The decisive factor is the effect of the behavior, one way or the other.

I'll give you an example. There was a businessman who was in two different courses with me, and then his wife was in a course. Somewhat later, she wrote me a letter saying that her husband had strangled his eighty-year-old mother and turned himself into the police. She asked me if I could help him. I told her that, for the sake of the dignity of the victim, I would be prepared to help him to face the consequences of his guilt.

I was called in by the police to give a statement that the man was not of sound mind. I refused. During the legal proceedings, it also came out that his adopted child had been killed in an accident. The man was freed, out of pity, because he was not of sound mind.

I told his wife that she had to get a divorce from him, that she couldn't stay with him. You can't stay with a murderer.

180

One day, he showed up at my door accusing me. I supposedly should have recognized that he was so aggressive. I told him that he belonged in prison, and that prison would be a place of dignity for him. I said that if he wasn't in prison, he should behave as if he were. He was very angry with me and left.

After a while I heard that since he was so wealthy, he had set up a foundation. He was a businessman and of perfectly sound mind. He named the foundation after his dead adoptive son, not after his mother. She was totally excluded.

A few weeks ago, I heard that his wife had committed suicide rather mysteriously. That's what comes of pity.

FRITZ I have anxiety attacks.

HELLINGER Since when?

FRITZ For about a year.

HELLINGER What happened at that time?

FRITZ I split up with my girlfriend.

HELLINGER Did something happen between you?

FRITZ No.

HELLINGER How are the anxiety states manifested?

FRITZ I have a horror of talking to people.

HELLINGER I had that, too, for thirty years. I got used to it and then forgot about it. *Fritz laughs.* Now, close your eyes, and imagine you're talking to someone, in a situation that makes you anxious. Feel the horror. When you feel it, pay attention to how old you are when you feel this.

After a while as Fritz makes an involuntary movement So, how old are you?

FRITZ *shaking his head* It seems like I wasn't even there. As if I'm not even here.

HELLINGER That could be. Did anything happen to your mother during the pregnancy?

FRITZ I don't know. My parents are already dead.

HELLINGER Did you ever hear anything, about an accident or anything?

FRITZ No, I don't know of anything.

HELLINGER We'll set up you and your mother. Choose representatives and place them.

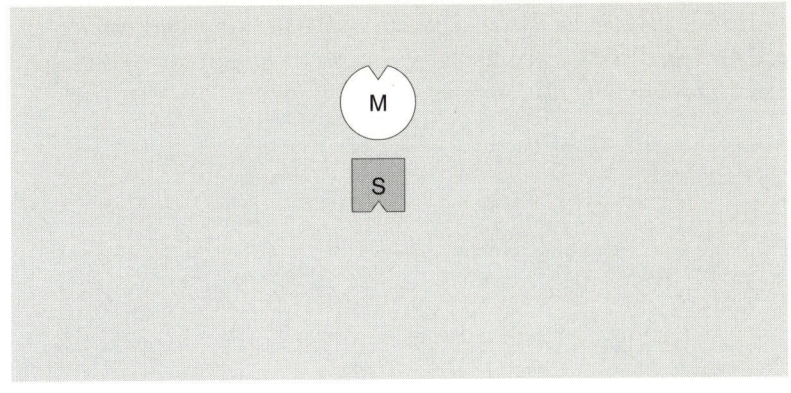

M   Mother
S   **Son (Fritz)**

The two representatives stand motionless for a while. Then, the mother's representative turns around and puts her hands on her son's back. She steps in front of him. They embrace warmly and the mother strokes her son's head.

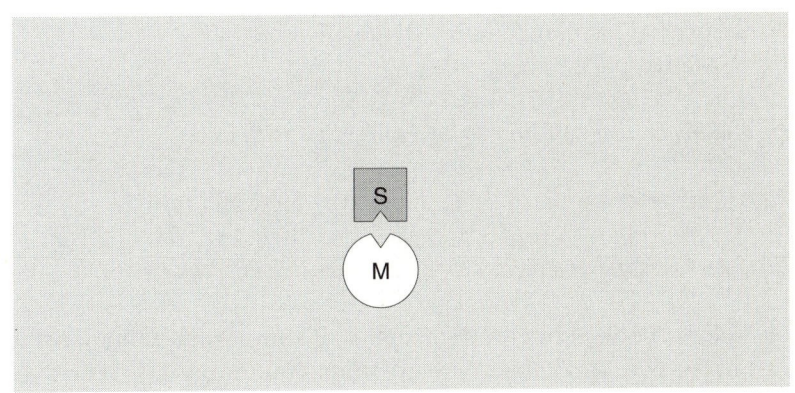

HELLINGER *after a while, to Fritz* How do you feel when you look at this?
FRITZ I'm shaking inside. I can't really believe it.
HELLINGER Go and stand there yourself.
To Fritz's representative How was that for you?
SON I couldn't turn around myself. I was afraid of all the people. Someone else had to take the initiative.

Fritz takes his place in the constellation and he and his mother embrace each other firmly. After a while, Hellinger chooses a representative for the father and brings him into the constellation.

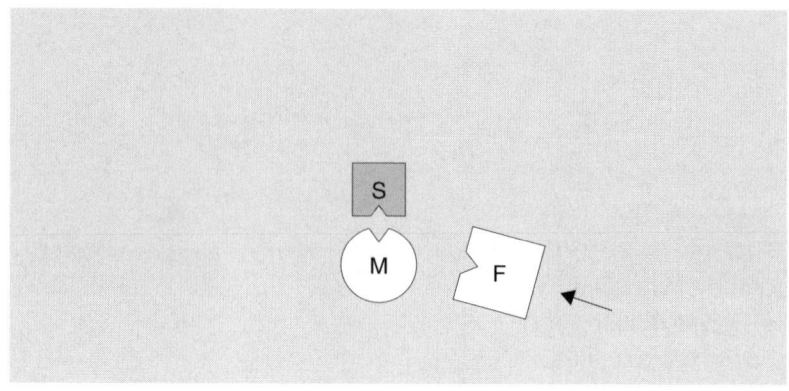

F   Father

After a short while, Fritz begins to sob.

HELLINGER *to Fritz* Say to her, "Mama, please stay."
FRITZ Mama, please stay.

He and his mother continue to hold each other with feeling.

HELLINGER *after a while, to Fritz* How are you doing now?

Fritz keeps crying and sighs deeply. He is unable to speak.

HELLINGER Look at her. With anxieties, it's important to look some-one in the eye. Anxieties come up when you look away. When you feel anxious, imagine you're looking into your mother's eyes.

He looks at his mother's representative and laughs.

HELLINGER You see? There it is.

Fritz and his mother continue to embrace. He gives her a kiss on the cheek. Hellinger then places the father's representative next to the mother's and moves Fritz to a place facing the two of them.

184

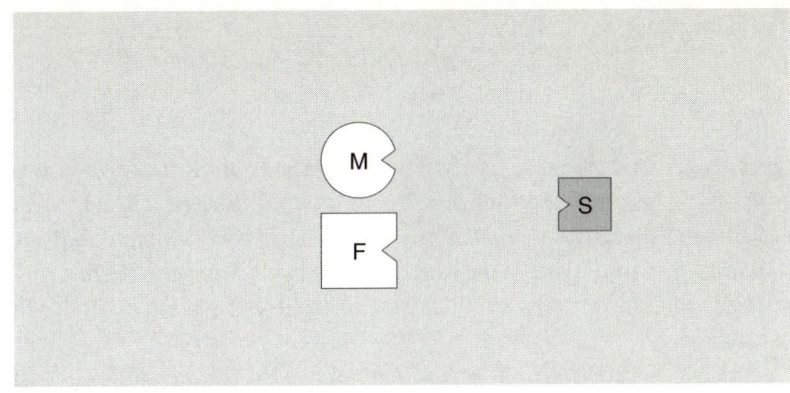

HELLINGER *to Fritz* Now look your father in the eye, too.

Fritz looks at his father and laughs.

HELLINGER I think that does it for you, right?
FRITZ Right.

FEAR

Once there was a man who went off to war. He had volunteered, got himself a machine gun, and went off to battle as a proud warrior. The enemy attacked and drew closer. In the army, there's a basic principle that you shouldn't fire until you see the whites of their eyes. Anybody can just fire a gun blindly, but it takes strength to wait until you see the whites of the enemy's eyes.

So, the enemy came closer and the man could see the whites of their eyes. He wanted to shoot, but he couldn't. His gun jammed. He began to tremble. As the enemy approached, he recognized him as his friend.

THE TURNING POINT
Rheumatoid arthritis and suicidal feelings

HELLINGER What is going on with you?

ELEANOR I've had rheumatoid arthritis for seven years. A year and a half ago, when my younger sister died, it was so bad that I was completely incapacitated. I was aware of wanting to follow her, even though I hadn't heard about you or your work at that time. She left me your book, *Zweierlei Glück*[1] and I decided to have a look at what was in it because I've also felt suicidal for about fifteen years.

HELLINGER That's enough. A while ago someone said that one effect of severe arthritis is that one can't go anywhere. *Eleanor nods.* Whatever going somewhere means. And sometimes, the illness leaves if the person stays.

ELEANOR *laughing* Since reading that book, I've decided to stay more firmly than I had in the past fifteen years. That's why I'm here.

HELLINGER Are you married?

ELEANOR I'm divorced.

HELLINGER Have you got any children?

ELEANOR No.

HELLINGER Why did you get divorced? I only mean the external reasons.

ELEANOR Actually, it was a long and happy marriage.

HELLINGER Did something happen?

ELEANOR There was another woman. But also, my husband made fun of my spiritual path, and I wasn't patient enough to be able to ride that out.

HELLINGER I make fun of that, too, sometimes.

ELEANOR Me too.

HELLINGER In the meantime?

ELEANOR I even enjoy doing it.

---

1 *Zweierlei Glück. Die systemische Psychotherapie Bert Hellingers*, ed. by Gunthard Weber, Heidelberg (Carl-Auer-Systeme Verlag) 1994, is also available in an English version as *Love's Hidden Symmetry. What Makes Love Work in Relationships*, ed. by Bert Hellinger with Gunthard Weber and Hunter Beaumont, Phoenix, AZ (Zeig, Tucker & Co) 1998.

HELLINGER I wouldn't go so far, myself. *Laughter in the group, Eleanor also laughs aloud.*

ELEANOR There's something else I'd like to say. My father was an alcoholic and committed suicide in a psychiatric hospital. Since then, I've been afraid of going crazy. His sister was also in a psychiatric clinic, and died there. That's been an underlying problem.

HELLINGER I'll start with you and your husband. Choose two representatives for you and him.

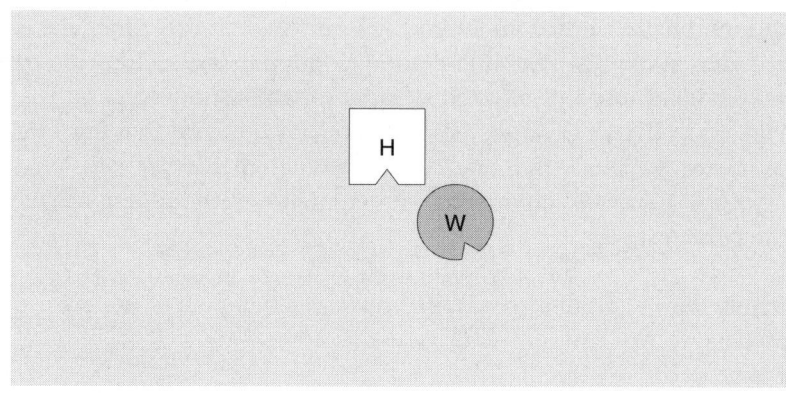

H   Husband
W   Wife (Eleanor)

The woman looks at the floor and the man shakes his head. After a while, he looks at her but she doesn't respond. She bows her head forward and is in danger of toppling over. Her husband takes her by the arm to hold her, but she doesn't react to him. He shakes his head again and lets go of her. He looks at her a while, then looks straight ahead.

HELLINGER *to Eleanor* What do you have to say about that?

ELEANOR (*crying, she indicates the constellation*) I'm very sad. I can't stand straight and firmly any more. My husband is simply there and he also gave me support. That's true, too.

HELLINGER There's no feeling for him there.

ELEANOR Yes. I feel, somehow, very sad, and I'm sorry about what I inflicted on him.

In the meantime, the husband is looking at his wife again.

188

HELLINGER The way you're talking, you're totally focussed on yourself, and you don't see your husband at all.

The husband's representative looks back at the floor and shakes his head. He looks at his wife again, shakes his head, and looks at the floor again. The woman remains motionless, but is dangerously close to falling over forward.

ELEANOR I see him.
HELLINGER That way you spoke about him was hardly sympathetic.
ELEANOR I'm also worried about him now.
HELLINGER What's that supposed to mean? What kind of worry about him? Looking at the picture that this constellation presents, it's arrogant to talk about worrying about him.

Hellinger places the two representatives facing one another.

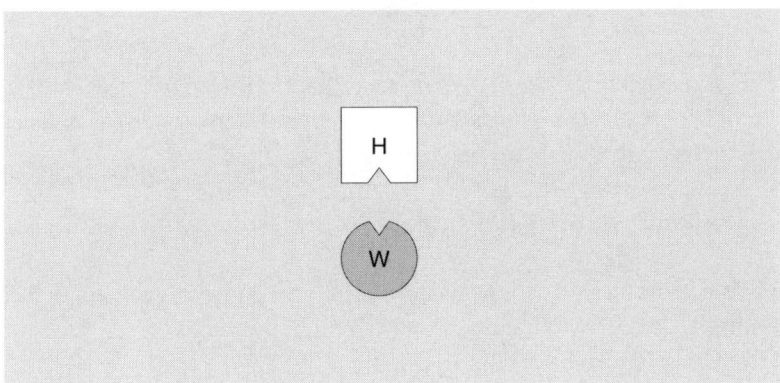

The man smiles at his wife in a friendly way, but she continues staring at the floor.

HELLINGER *to Eleanor* He is friendly, and she is closed.

The man shakes his head, looks at the floor and then at his wife again.

ELEANOR That's not true.
HELLINGER We can see it. We can see it here. That's what's presented to us. The disregard for a person is the beginning of a spiritual path. That's pictured here.

189

ELEANOR I don't exactly understand.

HELLINGER You talk too much instead of letting yourself be touched by the image.

The husband's representative takes a step backward. The wife also steps backwards and looks at her husband.

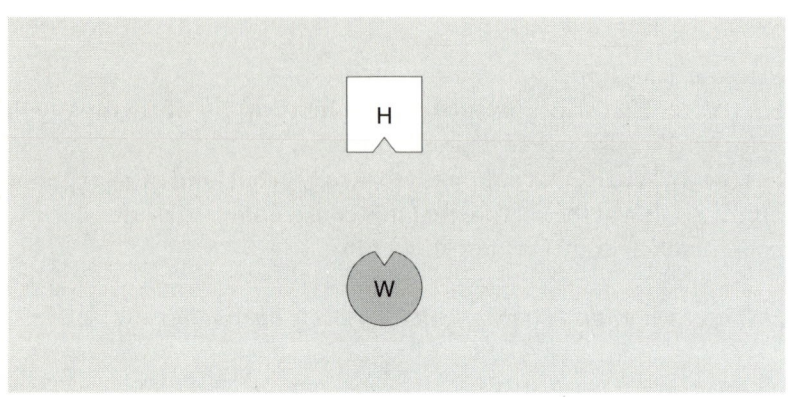

The only way out for the man is to leave. Never mind another woman! It's the only way out that allows him to keep his self-respect and his independence given what's coming from you.

The husband's representative nods.

HUSBAND It's over. It just won't work any more. I've waited long enough.

HELLINGER There's nothing to do.

HUSBAND I need to turn around.

HELLINGER Yes, do that.

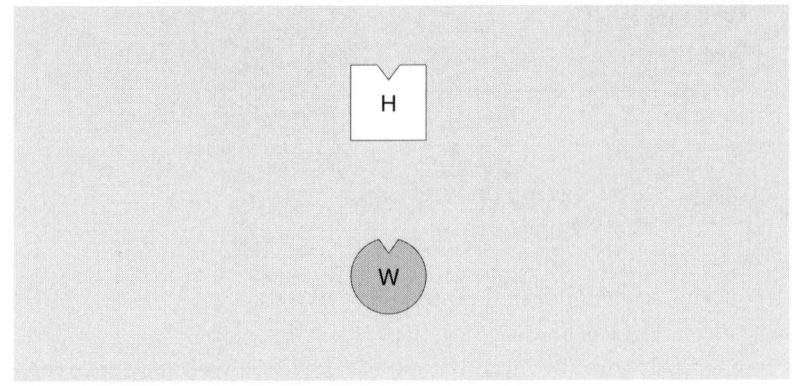

HELLINGER *to the representatives* You can both sit down.

After a while, to Eleanor, who is crying The turning point begins with a respect for your husband. *Eleanor nods.* Then you can look further. Okay?

ELEANOR Yes.

HELLINGER Okay. I'll leave it.

To group She clearly offered me the opportunity to look at her family of origin. That would have been a substitution.

To Eleanor You have to begin with the present. When that is resolved, you can go back to the family of origin and resolve what remains there.

To group Any questions?

PARTICIPANT I wouldn't have considered a spiritual path to be so bad. Earlier, when you were talking about phenomenology, I thought that perhaps that's something like a spiritual path.

HELLINGER *regards her closely for a long time* There is another path. It comes from on high back down to the earth.

HELLINGER What's going on with you?

CHARLOTTE I have breast cancer.

HELLINGER Since when?

CHARLOTTE I was operated on ten months ago.

HELLINGER How are you doing now?

CHARLOTTE Under the circumstances, I'm doing well. I've recovered well.

HELLINGER What would you like from me?

CHARLOTTE If possible, I'd like to get some support for believing and trusting that I can stay healthy. I'm afraid that I'll get ill again, that it will continue.

HELLINGER With some reason. Just imagine that you were convinced now that you would always remain healthy. How would you feel?

CHARLOTTE That would be totally unrealistic, I understand that.

HELLINGER It would also be terrible. For your soul it wouldn't be a good thing. The thing for you to do would be to take your illness to heart and deal with it with care, with respect, and with fear.

I did this fantasy with one of the first cancer patients I ever worked with. She was asked to imagine the cancer, until she had some image of it. She saw an octopus with many tentacles. Then I asked her to listen to what the octopus said. The octopus said, "Don't you know how dangerous I am?" The woman was confronted with the reality. That was many years ago. She's still alive. But that is the attitude that's called for. Pay attention to the danger too.

CHARLOTTE I know how dangerous this disease is.

HELLINGER Yes. I have a very simple picture. Set up a representative for cancer, and you stand next to it.

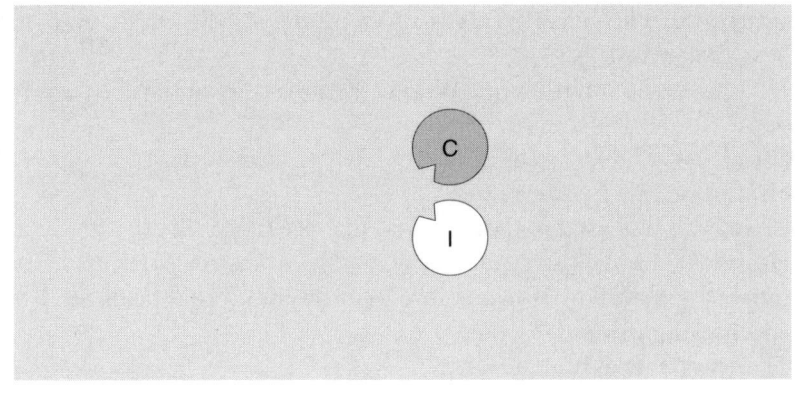

I Illness
C **Charlotte**

HELLINGER *to Charlotte, as she stands next to the representative of cancer*
Take her by the hand.

The representative of her cancer looks at Charlotte, who is breathing deeply and crying. Then Charlotte stands facing the cancer.

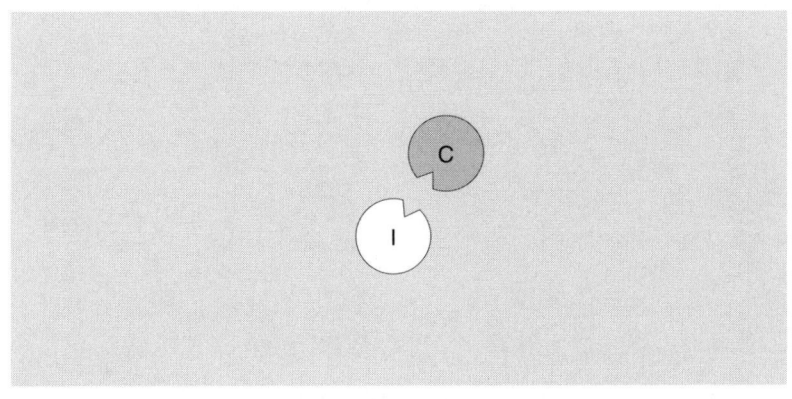

The two look at each other for a long time. The representative of cancer nods in a friendly way. After a while, Charlotte goes to the illness and they embrace. Charlotte is very moved. Then, they release their embrace and look at each other again.

HELLINGER Okay, that's good.
To Charlotte and the representative of her illness You two have demon-

strated this very nicely. This is also a model for the others here, for how to handle this.

I have one other image. Who is the illness, really? Who could it be?

CHARLOTTE I haven't a clue.

HELLINGER I saw your mother.

CHARLOTTE Yes, that makes sense to me. *She is very emotional.*

HELLINGER I have often noticed many breast cancer patients would rather die than bow down before their mother. What heals are love and bowing down.

To Charlotte Is that okay, now?

CHARLOTTE Yes.

THE DEAD NEED RESOLUTION
Two aborted children

HELLINGER What is it?
HEIDI It's my relationship.
HELLINGER What's happened?
HEIDI When I was 19 I got pregnant after a one-night stand. I had an abortion. While I was still pregnant, I met someone, and we fell in love. *She begins to cry.*
HELLINGER What happened?
HEIDI We were going to get married, and then I had a bad motorcycle accident and we split up.
HELLINGER What happened in the accident?
HEIDI I had a third-degree open break in my lower leg, but they were able to save the leg. Then, about four years ago, the scar opened up again. At that point, I did a family constellation of my family of origin with a therapist. The wound has slowly healed up again.

After that relationship, I was together with a man for twelve years, and I got pregnant again. There were medical reasons for terminating the pregnancy. After that, I gained a lot of weight. I had had that tendency before this, but this time it got really bad.
HELLINGER And what should I do? *After a while, when she doesn't answer* I'll tell you what makes someone get fat. You get fat when there's something missing. What's missing?
HEIDI A man.
HELLINGER No, two children are missing.
After a long silence Okay, set up representatives for you and for the two children.

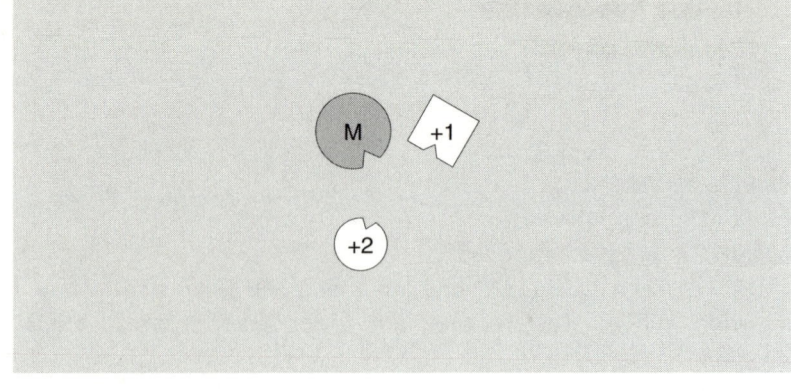

M   **Mother (Heidi)**
+1   First Aborted Child, a son
+2   Second Aborted Child, a daughter

Hellinger gives no instructions to the representatives. The representative of the first aborted child stares at the floor and begins to breathe heavily, shuddering as though he is going to throw up. The mother looks only at the aborted daughter.

Hellinger turns the mother's head to look at the aborted son. As they look at each other, the child's movements increase. The mother turns to him and puts her arm around him. The son moves closer to her and leans against her sobbing heavily. They embrace and hold each other tightly. The son's sobbing increases, and then he quiets down. Every so often he looks at her, but returns immediately to the embrace. Then, the mother and son take hands and the child sinks to the floor, kneeling before her with his arms around her knees, pressing his head against her. He then crouches down, pulling himself together, then holds her around the knees again. Finally, he stands up and embraces her.

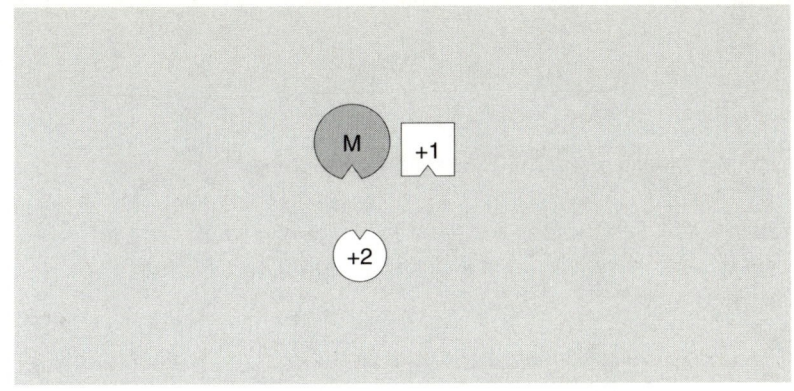

The mother then moves with the son towards her daughter She remains motionless for a while. The mother pets her head and pulls her to her. Then the daughter also puts her arm around her mother and all three embrace.

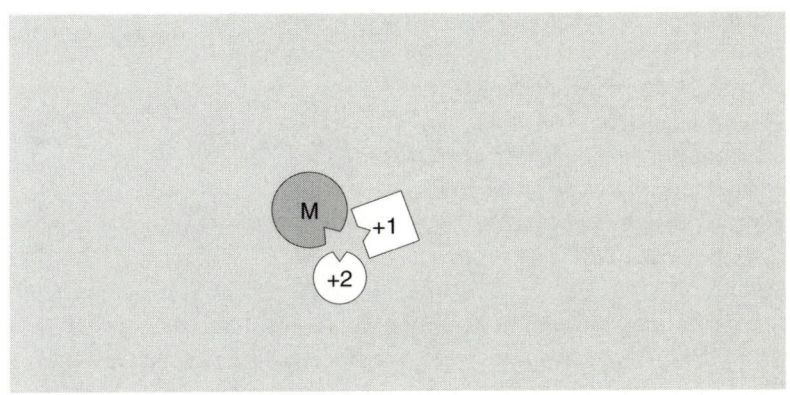

HELLINGER *to representatives* Okay, we'll leave it there. Thank you, all three of you.
To Heidi Is that all right with you?

Heidi nods.

HELLINGER *to group* The dead very often seem to need resolution. In this case you could see what that means.
After a long silence I'll tell you a story. You may have heard this story already, but in this context it takes on a special meaning.

One night a man dreamed he heard the voice of God telling him,

"Arise and take your only son, your beloved son, and lead him up onto the mountain which I will choose for you. There, kill him as a sacrifice to me."

The next morning the man awoke and looked at his only son, his only, beloved son. He looked at his wife, the mother of his son, and he looked at God.

He took the child up onto the mountain, built an altar, bound his son's hands, and pulled out his knife, ready to kill the boy. Just then he heard a different voice, and he killed a sheep instead.

How did the son look at his father?
How did the father look at his son?
How did the woman look at her husband?
How did the man look at his wife?
How did they look at God?
And, how did God – if he exists – look at them?

A different man dreamed in the night that he heard the voice of God telling him, "Arise and take your only son, your beloved son, and lead him up onto the mountain, which I will choose for you. There, kill him as a sacrifice to me."

The next morning the man awoke and looked at his only son, his only, beloved son. He looked at his wife, the mother of his son, and he looked at God. He answered God to his face, "No, I won't do that!"

How did the son look at his father?
How did the father look at his son?
How did the woman look at her husband?
How did the man look at his wife?
How did they look at God?
And, how did God – if he exists – look at them?

A PLACE
Breast cancer

HELLINGER *to Maria* Are you ready?
MARIA Yes.
HELLINGER What is going on with you?
MARIA I had a malignant breast tumor.
HELLINGER And how is it now?
MARIA It's been removed, and I'm hoping that I've overcome the illness and can keep overcoming it.
HELLINGER You can invite it into your bed to lie with you.
MARIA Into my bed with me?
HELLINGER You can invite the illness to lie in your bed with you. How would that be? *Maria is astounded and laughs.* Just imagine it. Close your eyes.

Maria becomes very calm and collected.

HELLINGER *as she makes as if to turn to him* Take your time, I'll give you all the time you need.

She closes her eyes again and remains very collected. After a while, Hellinger gently bows her head slightly forward. She bows her head deeper, shakes her head once and then breathes deeply.

HELLINGER *after a while* So, how is this illness as a bed partner?
MARIA She takes up a lot of room.
HELLINGER Okay, then we need a little more time. Continue with the exercise.

She closes her eyes again and bows her head deeply.

HELLINGER She is allowed to sleep with you in your bed.

After a while, Maria begins to breathe deeply again.

HELLINGER Give her as much room as she demands. *After a while* How old is she, then, lying by you?

199

MARIA *hesitating* Thirty-five. *(Maria's age)*
HELLINGER Okay, just continue.

She closes her eyes again and sits quietly for a long time. Every now and then she sighs deeply and straightens up.

HELLINGER What's happening now?
MARIA At first she lay over me like a blanket. Now she's rolled herself up at the end of the bed, like a rolled up blanket.
HELLINGER Yes. That's what happens when you give her a place.
MARIA Will she stay lying there now? *She laughs.*
HELLINGER She'll remain there unless you chase her away. Then she'll spread out.
MARIA I feel very fearful seeing that.
HELLINGER You've forgotten that you were at the brink of death.
MARIA Yes, that's true.
HELLINGER You can't ever forget that. You have to give that a place, now. And your life will have a deeper level of meaning.

She is overcome with emotion and closes her eyes again.

MARIA *after a while* That feels good.
HELLINGER Yes. That's it then.

200

FATHER AND SON
Addiction

HELLINGER *to Luther* What is the issue with you?

LUTHER My problem is that I have a strong sense that I'm not living my own life. It feels as if there were some kind of strange being inside of me holding me back. It's something I have no defense against. I feel like if I don't get rid of it, I haven't got a chance. *Full of emotion:* When I look back at my life it seems like everything I've done has gone down this destructive path, and I can't change any of that, either.

HELLINGER What do you mean by destructive paths?

LUTHER Even as a little kid, six years old, I had suicidal fantasies. Later, I started drinking a lot and ended up with multiple drug dependency. I also attempted suicide several times, twice when I was twenty, and once more about six years ago. I went into therapy at that point and things seemed to get better for a while. Now, for a while, the old things have been slipping in again.

HELLINGER Are you married?

LUTHER No, I'm single.

HELLINGER Have you got any children?

LUTHER No, not that, either.

HELLINGER What happened in your family of origin?

LUTHER From what I know of my mother's family, her eldest brother went missing in Russia, that is, he never came back from the war. My grandfather on my father's side was a doctor and in the SS. At the end of the war when it was clear that everything was going to collapse, he poisoned himself and everyone in his family except my father.

HELLINGER That's enough.

Luther is crying and closes his eyes. He then tries to bring his feelings under control.

HELLINGER Stay with your feelings and look at all the dead.

Hellinger indicates to a man in the group to come up and stand behind Luther, who is sitting next to Hellinger.

HELLINGER *to this representative* Put your hands on his shoulders. You are his father.

Luther covers his face and is crying hard.

HELLINGER *after a while, to Luther* Imagine that here in front of you there's your grandfather, and all the poisoned people, and behind them lie the other victims of your grandfather. Look at them all.

Luther looks and continues crying. Then, he shuts his eyes again.

HELLINGER Really look at them. Take your time and look at them. Slowly move from one to another, and allow them to look at you too.

The father's representative behind Luther is becoming very restless and looks away.

HELLINGER *to the representative* You can't look at them? Then lie down with them.

He lies down on his back in front of Luther.

HELLINGER *to Luther* He turned away. Your father couldn't look at them. Tell your father, "I'll look for you."
LUTHER I'll look for you.
HELLINGER And look at them.
LUTHER *after a while* I feel drawn to the dead.
HELLINGER Exactly. Imagine for a moment that you were lying down with them. Just imagine it, though. Look at them and imagine yourself lying with them, with love and respect.

Hellinger goes to the father's representative on the floor and turns his head to one side, facing away from Luther.

HELLINGER *to father's representative* Turn towards the dead and close your eyes.

The father's representative sobs.

HELLINGER *after a while to Luther* How are you feeling now?
LUTHER There's a feeling of relief, and a desire to go to my father.
HELLINGER Go to him.

Luther lies down next to his father. He puts his arms around him and lays his head on his father's chest. The father continues looking away towards the dead. They remain like that for a long time. Then, the father looks over at his son.

HELLINGER Now both of you stand up.

They stand up next to one another, with their arms around each other.

HELLINGER *to the father's representative* How is that for you, now?
FATHER I feel like I'm looking for him too. I'm getting strong. I want things to be okay for him. Looking at the dead gave me strength. Before, I just wanted to get away, but when I heard him talking, I realized that I had to look there. I want to protect him and take over whatever I have to.
HELLINGER *to Luther* And for you, now?
LUTHER I get a lot of strength from him being here with me, close to me, and from his support.

Father and son laugh together.

LUTHER It's like there's something there that was never there before.
HELLINGER Okay, I think we'll leave it there.
LUTHER *laughing* Yes, thanks.

HELLINGER *to Katja* What's the issue?

KATJA Seven years ago, my husband and my son both committed suicide within three months of each other. I still can't really let the pain of that in.

HELLINGER Most of all, because you're angry with them.

KATJA I'm not angry, I often look ...

HELLINGER When the pain doesn't stop, there's anger there. When you lose someone you really love, after a while the pain is finished. But, if you're angry with that person, for example, because he killed himself, then the pain doesn't go away. It's also not a pain for the other person, it's a pain for yourself, and there's no resolution. What would you say to that?

KATJA I'd have to look at it from that viewpoint first.

HELLINGER We'll set up a constellation with three people: your husband, your son, and you. Choose three representatives and place them in relation to each other.

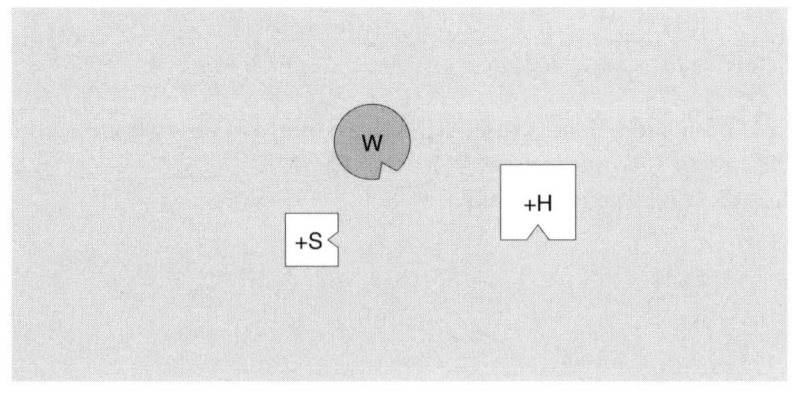

W	Wife (Katja)	+S	Son
+H	Husband		

The son stares continually at the floor.

HELLINGER *after a while, to Katja's representative* How are you feeling?

WIFE I feel like a spectator in the middle of what's going on here.
HELLINGER That's right.

Hellinger moves her back further.

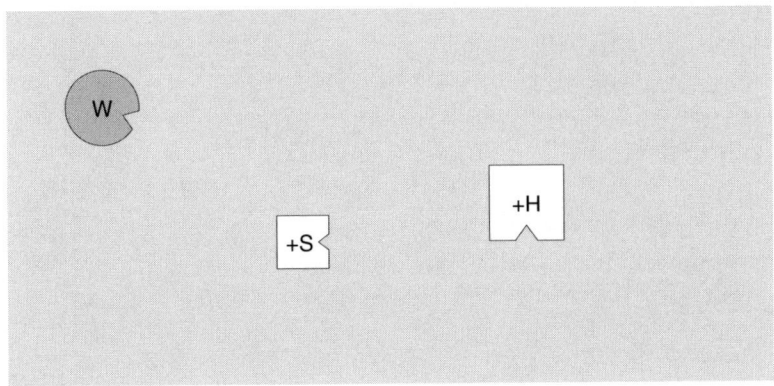

HELLINGER How is that?
WIFE That's better. This way I can see them both.

Hellinger turns her away.

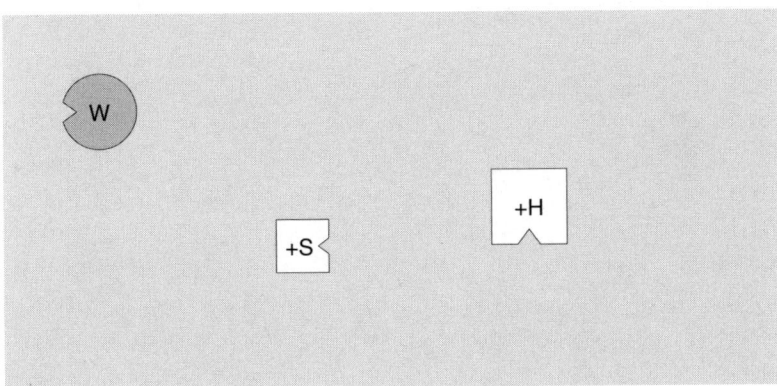

HELLINGER How is that?
WIFE I can't see anything anymore, but, *(sighs)* actually it's good like this.
HELLINGER Exactly.
To Katja That's the resolution. You can't get involved.

HELLINGER *to husband's representative* What's going on with you?
HUSBAND I don't feel well. I don't know what's going on behind me.
Strange.

Hellinger turns him towards his wife and son.

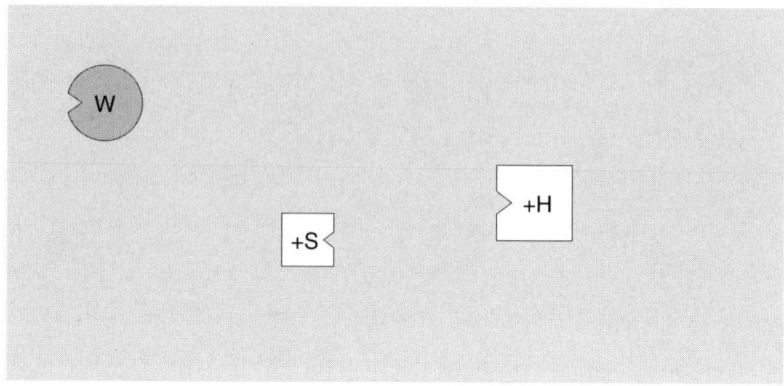

HELLINGER How is that?
HUSBAND I can't do anything with that.

Hellinger turns him away from the others again.

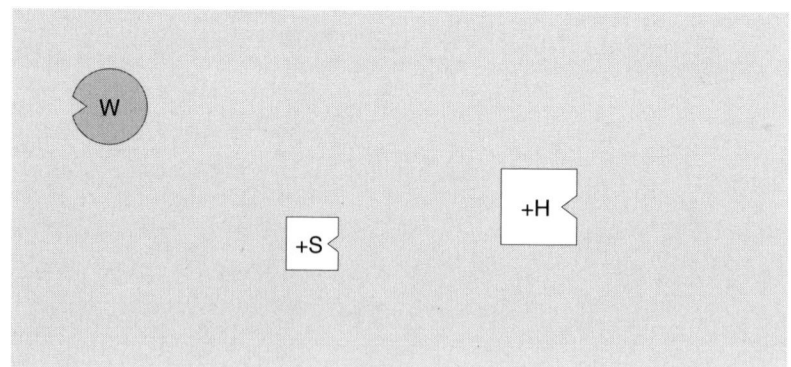

HELLINGER How is that?
HUSBAND There's a certain relief.
HELLINGER *to son* And for you?
SON It's terrible. I feel totally unprotected, observed, like I'm naked.
I just want to sink through the floor ... to be dead ... to be gone.

206

Hellinger leads him to his father. He moves with his head and arms hanging. Then, he lays his head on his father's chest, and the father puts his arm around him. The son sobs.

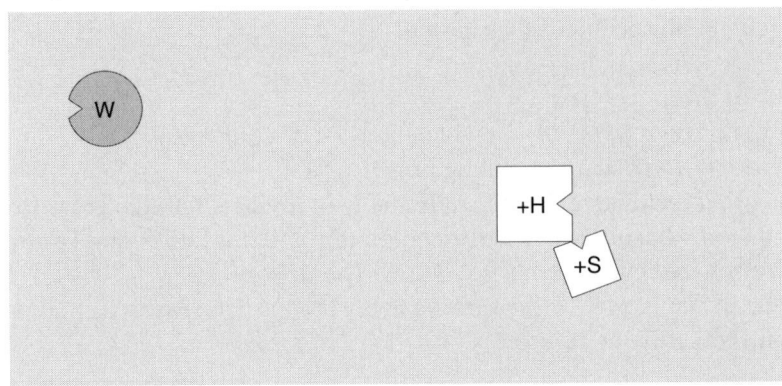

HELLINGER *after a while, to Katja's representative* Turn around again, so you can see them.

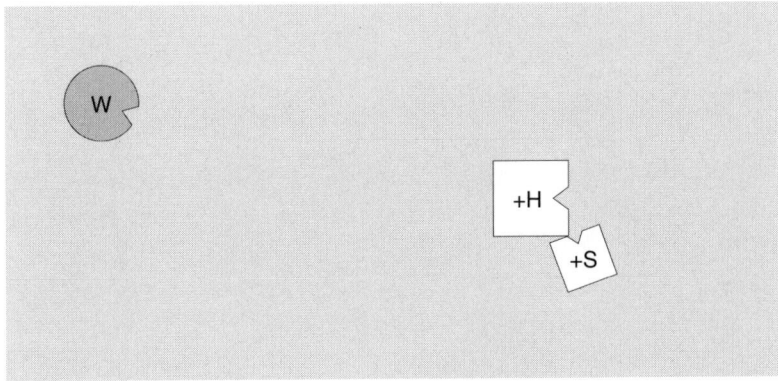

WIFE *after a while* That was important for me. Somehow I could feel that there was something going on there, but that I couldn't have any part in it.

HELLINGER *to son* How are you doing, now?

SON *sighs* I feel sort of taken care of. It's warm here and I can hear his heart beating. That's good.

HELLINGER *to Husband* And for you?

HUSBAND It's better, yes.

HELLINGER *to group* In a situation like this there's something important to be considered. It appears as though we might be able to influence the dead, in good ways and in bad ways. If you don't let the dead go, it's bad for them. No matter what was going on there, together, they will find their peace.

To Katja Is that okay for you?

KATJA Yes.

HELLINGER *to representatives* Now get out of your roles.

To Katja How are you feeling now?

KATJA I feel better. That's really the way it was. I felt like I was in a cinema. My son wanted to be completely with his father, and I didn't want to believe that. It's good now. Thank you.

HELLINGER And now the turning away is complete. Away from them and towards the future.

HELLINGER *to group* When it comes to suicide, survivors often have the feeling that they could have prevented it. They feel guilty about it, often, as if they have killed the person. But, someone who commits suicide kills himself, or herself. That can't ever be pushed off onto another person. We don't know what influences are working in the background. It is almost always an entanglement of some kind.

Someone's fate may have its roots far back in the family history, sometimes many generations. If this fate of a deceased person is not respected in the family, then someone in the following generation may feel an inexplicable pressure to commit suicide. They have no idea why.

If the mother or father of a family die young, their children often feel drawn to follow the parent into death. Or, sometimes when a child senses that one of the parents is drawn towards death, the child says, "I'll do it instead of you."

There are often similar circumstances in a couple relationship. When one of the partners feels the other partner's pull towards suicide, he or she does it instead. The basis is a deep love and honor, but it's totally unconscious.

For anyone who feels suicidal, it's a healing exercise to go to the other dead in the family. The person imagines that they are sinking into the realm of the dead and lying next to the others who have died. It's like an anticipatory suicide, if you like. The person goes to the dead and stays there with them for a while, waiting. As a rule, some sign comes from the dead, or a strength that serves life. The person has to open his or her heart to this offering and then return to the living. It's a healing exercise.

On the other hand, some are drawn to the dead in the fantasy that the dead will benefit from this act. They don't attend to what comes from the dead. That has bad effects. And then, there are those who remain constantly with the dead in their thoughts.

To Katja That's what you were doing. You were living with the dead instead of the living, and that's not good.

There is an inner conflict between really seeing and the images we hold for ourselves, of our feelings and hopes and fears. Really looking takes away the fear. That's the first thing. Someone in a highly emotional state who takes the time to really look will notice a change in the feelings. They resolve into something less complicated.

This is the work of the therapist, to lead the client to a place of looking and really seeing, independent of all the inner pictures, fears, hopes, or whatever. The therapist is also looking, and remains unaffected by the hopes, feelings, or fears of the client. Rather, he or she looks and sees what is actually true at that moment in time, and takes it very seriously.

When someone is worked up in a state of high emotion, they often close their eyes. The feelings are dependent on inner pictures, and that's why the person has to close their eyes. If they open their eyes, they can't maintain these images. Then, the feelings alter and you get to solid ground, where there's the possibility of movement.

ONE TRAGEDY IS ENOUGH
Manic depressive illness

HELLINGER *to Veronica* How are you feeling?

VERONICA I've been thinking about being ill. I am manic-depressive.

HELLINGER Do you know what manic means?

VERONICA Yes.

HELLINGER What does it mean?

VERONICA To be very high.

HELLINGER In the Heavens, that's what it means. In Heaven, you're dead, you know? Everyone who is in Heaven is dead. Wanting to go up to Heaven means wanting to die, and those who want to die, want to go up to Heaven, whichever way round you look at it. I see a connection between manic states and an identification with someone who is dead, and wanting to get to Heaven. Does that have any meaning for you?

Veronica nods energetically and begins to cry.

HELLINGER Let's look at the reality. I am real and you are real, so look at me. Now, who is the dead person?

VERONICA The dead person is my grandfather's first wife, on my mother's side.

HELLINGER What happened to her.

VERONICA She set fire to herself in the bathtub. *She sobs.*

HELLINGER Watch out. She's the one who did it. And what are you doing?

VERONICA I'm going to kill myself.

HELLINGER Look at her in the bathtub. *As Veronica refuses, shaking her head* You have to look. Haven't I just finished telling you about looking? *She laughs.* Exactly. You have to look them in the eye.

She looks calmly forward.

HELLINGER *after a while* That's what you can make out of despair.

Veronica nods and continues looking forward. Then, she drops her head and begins to cry again.

211

HELLINGER *after a while* Imagine you had been in the bathtub and had set fire to yourself. And then imagine that two generations down the line, someone comes along and wants to jump out of a window on your account. If you were aware of that, how would you feel in your bathtub?

VERONICA It wouldn't bother me.

HELLINGER Take a minute to really get into it. You weren't in that place when you answered.

She looks forward again.

HELLINGER Are you married? *She nods.* Have you got children? *She shakes her head, no.* Can you imagine having children? How it might be?

VERONICA I don't have any children because of the illness.

HELLINGER That's okay. Just imagine that you had children and grand-children, and you're standing at the window, ready to jump out. All of a sudden, you're aware that two generations later, someone is go-ing to set fire to himself in a bathtub, out of love for you. What hap-pens to you at the window?

VERONICA In that case, I wouldn't jump.

HELLINGER And if you decided to jump anyway, what would you say to your grandchild?

She considers this for a long time.

HELLINGER I can tell you. Shall I tell you? Yes? *She nods.* You'd say, "One tragedy is enough."

Veronica laughs and nods.

HELLINGER She would have undoubtedly said the same to you.

VERONICA Yes.

HELLINGER She's saying that to you now.

She bows her head and cries.

HELLINGER *after a while* I'm not an expert in the field, but I've been told that manic-depressive illness is curable. Okay?

VERONICA *laughing* Okay.

212

HELLINGER What is the issue?

FERDINAND At the moment, I don't know where to begin. We are at a real crisis point in our relationship. We have a three-year-old daughter. The birth was very difficult and she is quite severely handicapped.

HELLINGER What kind of handicap?

FERDINAND A so-called leukodystrophia. It's a kind of brain damage. The stuff called myelin is missing and that hinders her development, both physical and mental. The doctors have been unable to give us any prognosis about what will happen in the future. This child has been very demanding on us for the past three years. At first she had a cannula (a tube which allows the release of fluid) and she was more or less continuously in an intensive care unit at home, with medical attendants. In the meantime, she's doing better, but we have pulled apart from one another. I'm aware that we can't support each other emotionally very much. Most of all with the difficult feelings, the grief, abandonment, hopelessness. We can't share these and a terrible loneliness has developed.

HELLINGER *to Monica* Would you like to add anything to this?

MONICA This child was my fourth attempt to have a child, and it was successful. Before, with Ferdinand, I had two miscarriages. During this pregnancy, I was quite fearful of losing this baby, too. Actually, the feeling of distance between us has been growing ever since the first miscarriage. We both feel left alone in this relationship. Still, we would like to stay together.

HELLINGER We'll set up a representative only for this child.

To Monica Will you choose someone, please?

HELLINGER *to the child's representative* Have you ever seen a constellation, how it is done? *She nods.* Okay. First, collect yourself in this child in relationship to the parents. Then, just let happen whatever happens.

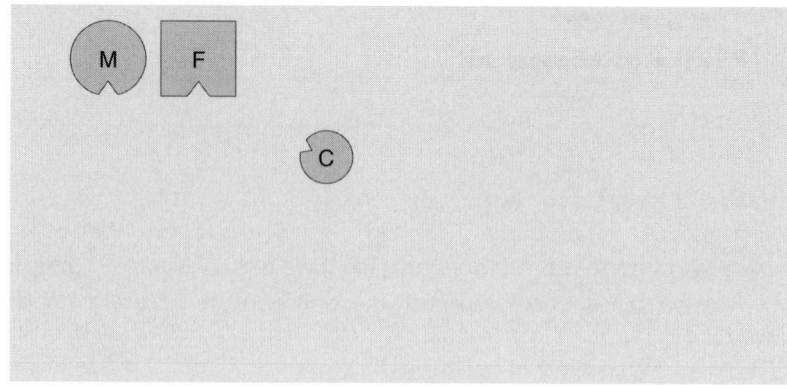

C   Child, a daughter, severely handicapped
F   **Father (Ferdinand)**
M   **Mother (Monica)**

The child's representative breathes deeply and stares at the floor, and then up at the two parents. After a while, Hellinger moves her a step backwards, away from the parents. He holds her arm as she continues to look at her parents. Then, he leads her still another few steps backwards, and then, after a while, a few more.

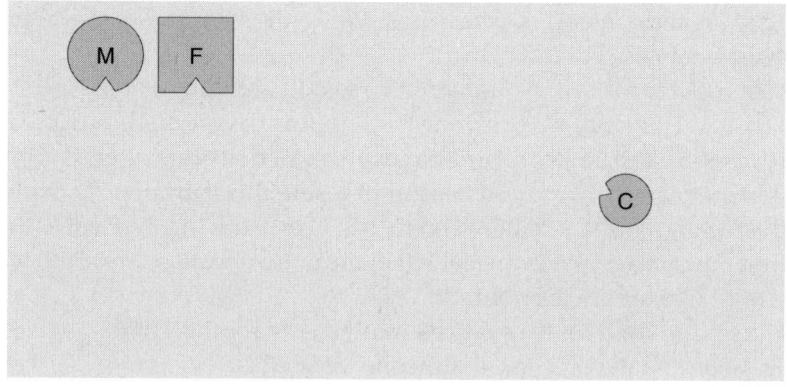

After a while, Hellinger chooses two representatives for the miscarried children and places them behind the handicapped child, who sobs aloud. One of the miscarried children stares only at the floor.

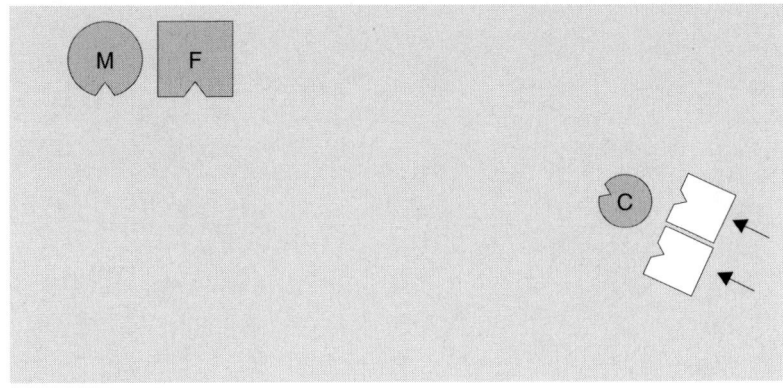

HELLINGER *after a while, to the handicapped child's representative* Turn around.

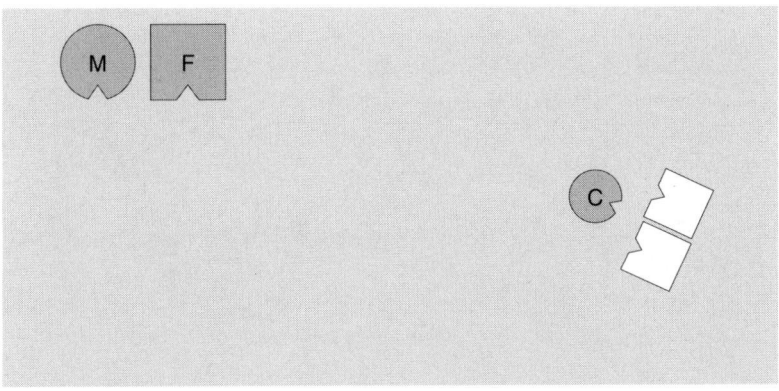

The handicapped child looks at the two miscarried children and weeps. Then everything is quieter. The miscarried children hold hands and put an arm around their sister. After a while, Hellinger moves the sister close to the other two children. The three embrace warmly. Hellinger calls the parents over and they also embrace all three children, with sobs.

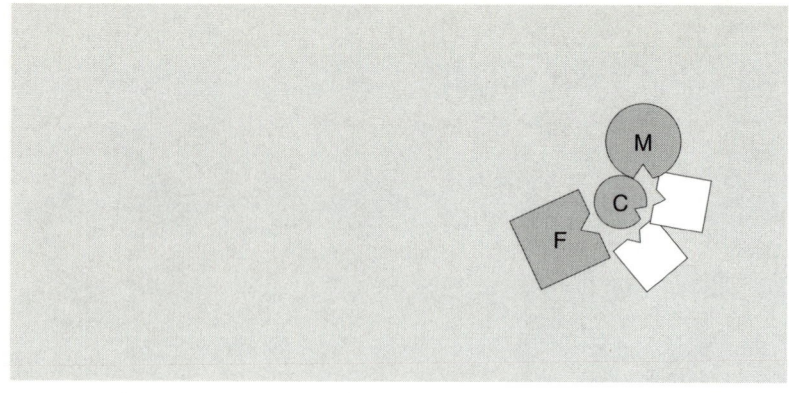

HELLINGER *after a while, to the representative of the handicapped child* Now turn around so you can see your parents, and lean against these two miscarried siblings.

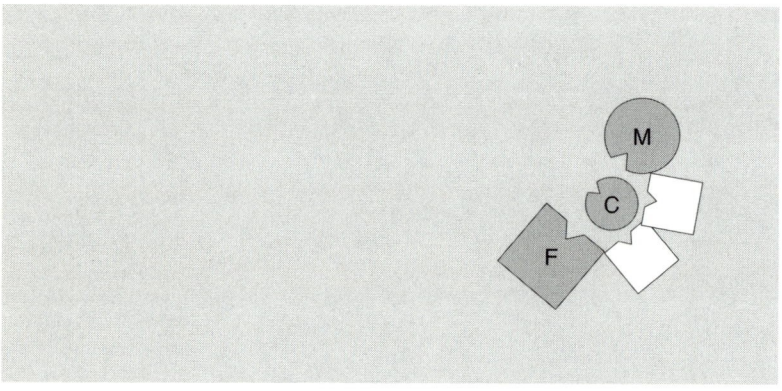

The handicapped child puts her arms around her mother and father. Then, all five form a group and embrace.

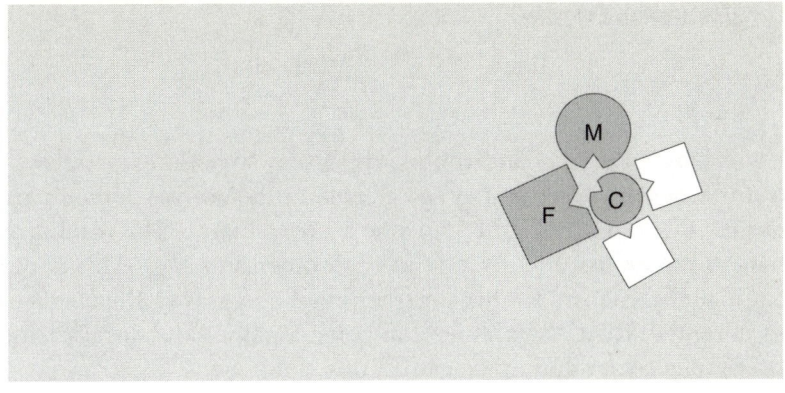

HELLINGER *after a while, to the handicapped child* How are you feeling?
CHILD Great.
HELLINGER And the mother?
MONICA I feel very supported. We're together.
HELLINGER The father?
FERDINAND I feel a lot of love, and I feel very connected.
HELLINGER *to Monica* Tell your husband, "This is our child."
MONICA This is our child.
HELLINGER *to Ferdinand* Look at your wife and say the same to her.
FERDINAND This is our child.

The representative of the handicapped child sobs heavily.

HELLINGER *to this child* Tell them, "You are my parents."
CHILD You are my parents.
HELLINGER We'll leave it there.

To Ferdinand and Monica When a man and a woman become a couple,
they are full of joy and look happily into the future. They are driven
by a force that brings them together. Whatever is behind, or beneath
this force, and this depth, and this love, and this demand, remains
hidden to you. It only slowly comes to light what it really means, as
it has with you just now. When you can connect to this driving force,
the foreground events seem insignificant. But you can find your way
back to each other out of this connection to that power and the depth.

When parents have a handicapped child, they sometimes move away from each other, because they secretly blame themselves or their partner for the handicap, as if someone were to blame. The resolution here is for the parents to look at each other and say, "This is our child, and we'll care for her together in whatever way she needs us as parents." Then, the parents can come together and support and strengthen each other in the care of this child.

Often, people outside feel sorry for the parents of a handicapped child, as if they have had really bad luck. If you look at these families, however, and see how they deal with a handicapped child, and if you really see what strength comes into the family in this way, then you can see that a handicapped child has a special meaning for a family. The strength of love, gentleness, and of discipline. The family of a handicapped child shines on those around them. Many illusions one might have about happiness and life dwindle and make way for a deep love of life as it is, even with its limitations.

When there are many miscarriages or stillbirths, or infant deaths in a family, it often leads to a separation of the parents. The resolution is for the parents to grieve together. When grief is permitted, love can flow. It demonstrates something about the greatness of parenthood, of having children and losing children, and still holding to each other.

"I'LL LEAVE YOU WITH YOUR PARENTS"
Abuse in the mother's family

HELLINGER *to Monica* Is there something unfinished from your family of origin? What happened there?

MONICA For example?

HELLINGER How many children were there?

MONICA Four.

HELLINGER Did any of them die?

MONICA No.

HELLINGER Were either of your parents in a serious relationship prior to their marriage?

MONICA No.

HELLINGER Are there any illegitimate children anywhere?

MONICA No.

HELLINGER What happened in your mother's family?

MONICA My grandparents, my mother's parents, are difficult for me and my mother.

HELLINGER What happened?

MONICA My grandmother was a very cold, distant woman, who had to fight for her life. My grandfather was a very unpredictable man who, I think, abused his daughter and, I believe, me as well. My grandmother had a lot of power over my mother.

HELLINGER That's enough. We'll set up a constellation of the grandmother, your mother and you. Choose three representatives.

When Monica has chosen her representatives, Hellinger places them.

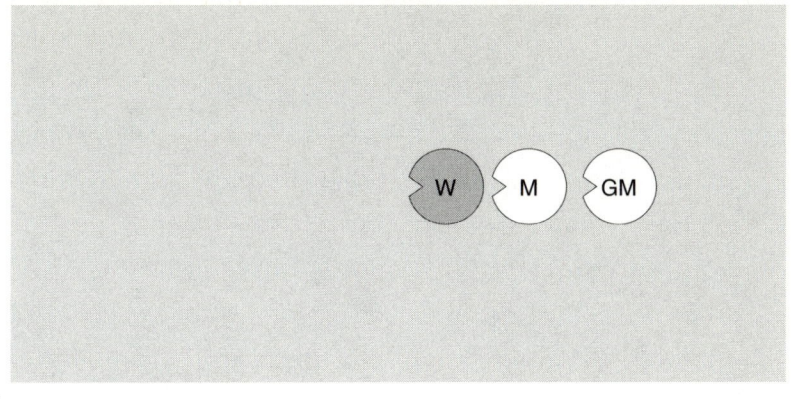

W **Woman (Monica)** GM Grandmother
M Mother

Monica's mother leans against the grandmother and Monica's representative leans against her mother. The representative for Monica's mother begins to shake. Hellinger chooses a representative for the grandfather and places him next to the grandmother.

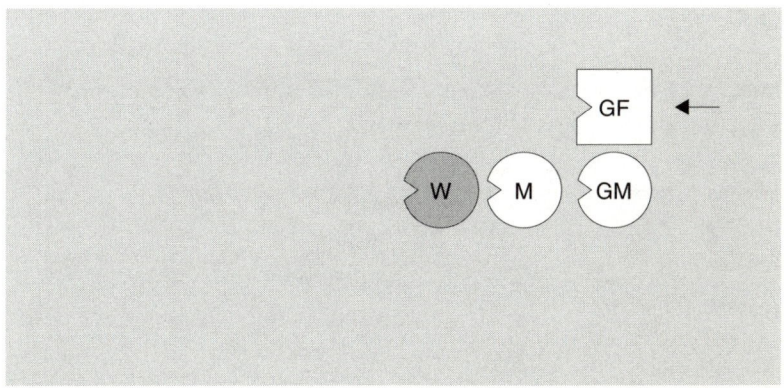

GF Grandfather

The mother's shaking increases. She is in danger of collapsing and falling over to the left. Her entire body is shaking and the others circle around her and hold her up. Hellinger leads Monica's representative further away. The grandparents continue holding the trembling mother. She then quiets down somewhat. Hellinger has her turn around to her parents and put her arms around them.

221

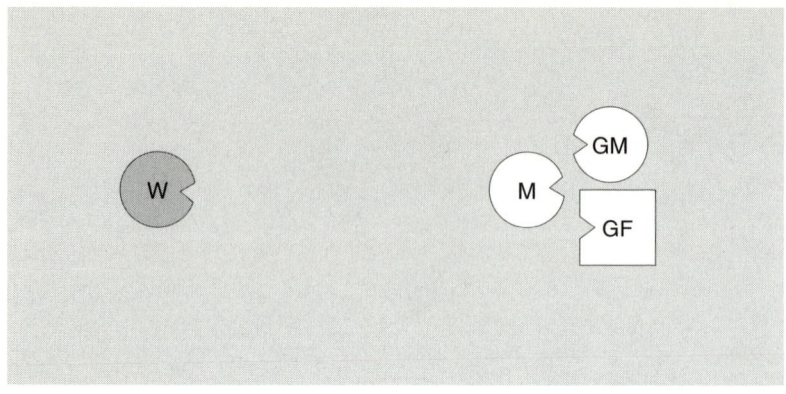

Monica's mother begins shaking again and screams loudly. The grandparents hold her tightly. She slowly calms down.

HELLINGER *after a while, to Monica's Mother* Now look at your parents and say to each of them, "Yes."

She looks at them for a long time, and after a hesitation she says "Yes" to each of them.

HELLINGER *to Monica's Mother* Now lean against your parents with your back to them, and look forward.

She leans back against them and they hold her shoulders.

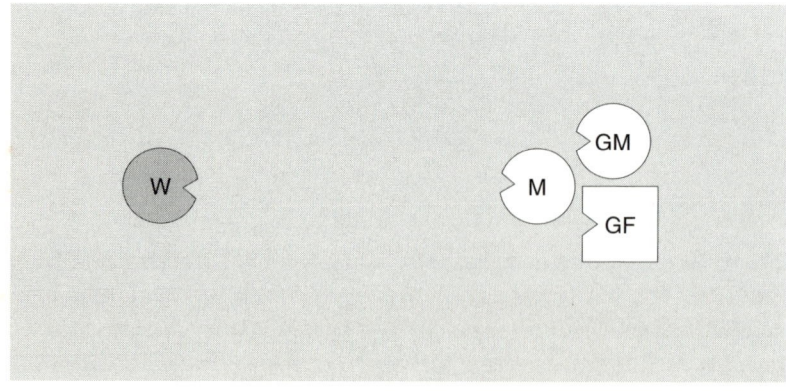

HELLINGER *to Monica's representative* How are you feeling now?

WOMAN Better over here at a distance. Before, my back was all cramped up. I don't feel like a part of this, though.

HELLINGER Tell your mother, "I'll leave you with your parents."

WOMAN I'll leave you with your parents.

Hellinger chooses a representative for Monica's father and places him in the constellation.

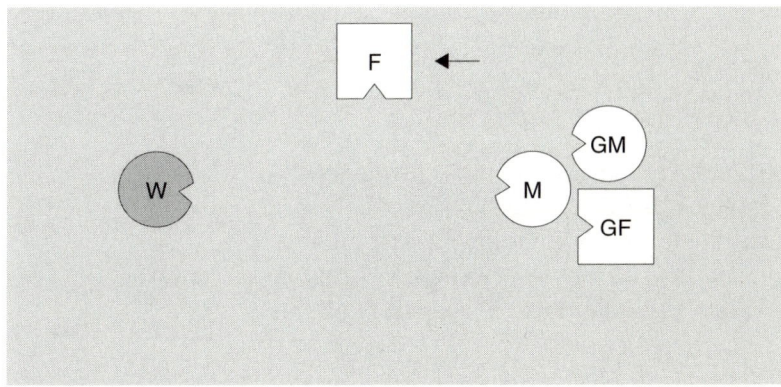

F   Father

HELLINGER *to Monica's Mother* How is that for you with him standing there?

MOTHER I'm not so sure. But now somebody's there. The barrier to my daughter isn't so great. As far as I'm concerned, she could come closer.

Hellinger moves Monica's father next to Monica's mother.

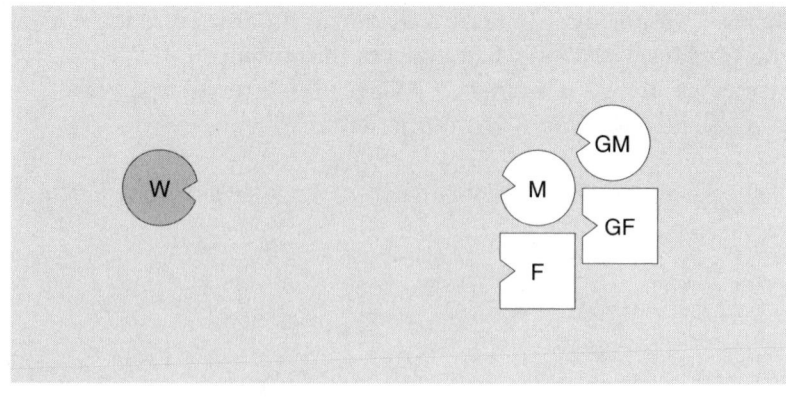

HELLINGER *to Monica's Mother* How is that?
MOTHER I like that better.
FATHER I'm meeting her for the first time.
HELLINGER *to Monica's representative* And for you now?
WOMAN I still don't feel like a part of all this.

Hellinger leads Monica's representative to her parents and has her lean back against them. After a while he brings in the representative of her handicapped child, from the previous constellation, and has her lean backwards against her mother.

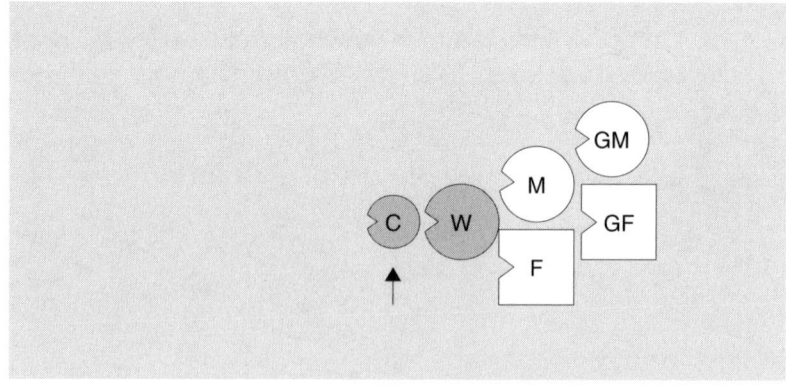

C   Child, a daughter, severely handicapped

HELLINGER *after a while, to Monica's representative* Follow your impulse.

Monica's representative bows her head down to the child and weeps. She puts her arms around her child from behind. Both are filled with emotion. The child leans back and lays her head on her mother's shoulder. She nestles back in and sighs deeply. After a while Hellinger has the child face her mother.

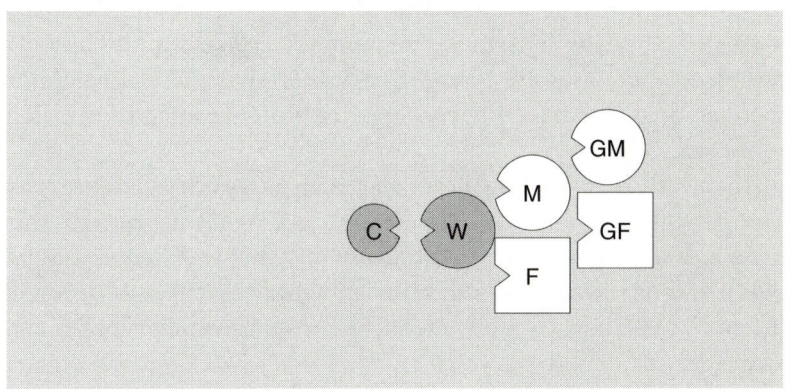

The child strokes her mother's cheek. They look at each other for a long time. The child laughs, and they take each other's hands. The mother breathes deeply.

HELLINGER Okay, that's all.
To Monica Is that okay for you?

Monica nods.

HELLINGER I would like to say a bit about remembering.

Traumatic events, such as child abuse, are often repressed so that they are no longer consciously remembered. Freud said that when repressed memories are brought back into awareness, a healing is then possible. But that is not enough. Just bringing something to light is not sufficient.

In addition, something is needed, such as we have just seen here. The person has to stand in agreement with what happened. They have to stand in agreement with the reality that was, without regret that it was as it was, and without wishing things had been different. If this can be done, then even terrible events become peaceful, with strength.

We have to let go of fantasies of well-being that we may have had before. The enormity is frightening, but if you can face it straight on and agree to it, something that has been previously hidden will come to light, and that something is an incredible love. That's the really strange thing.

To Monica Now look into your husband's face.

Ferdinand and Monica look at each other for a long time. Ferdinand nods to her and puts his arm around her. She puts a hand on his knee.

HELLINGER *to the couple* That's where we'll leave this. All the best to both of you.

To group Here, we have looked at many different levels of remembering. At first there were the miscarried children who were not remembered. We could see what happens when the dead who have been forgotten because it was too painful to remember them are allowed to be present. We have seen what happens when one is allowed to go to them. The dead are present. Otherwise they wouldn't have such a powerful effect on the living. They are present in some obscure way. We can acknowledge their presence by keeping company with them, perhaps even lying down with them.

To Monica and Ferdinand For example, you might imagine these children lying in bed between you. The peculiar thing is that after a while they'll leave that place. What is acknowledged and loved, pulls away after a while. When these children are recognized, a strength comes from them, which can give you strength for your handicapped child. That's one level of remembering.

Then, we had a second layer of memories of a grandfather who was a perpetrator. We don't need or want to go into the details of that. Perpetrators are often excluded from the heart. There is an exercise that helps in such a situation. If you look back at the course of your own life, each of you will come to some point where you were guilty of something, a point where you hurt someone, a point where you were a perpetrator. Often we don't want to admit this and we repress those memories. That becomes our shadow, which we deny.

If you can hold the knowledge of your own guilt, and the memories of the damage you have caused, and lie down with the dead perpetrator with this full awareness until you feel calm and at one with him, then there can be reconciliation. The perpetrator is reconciled because his evil is at an end when someone else lies down next to him. You are reconciled because, strangely enough, in being at one with the perpetrator, your own evil also comes to an end.

One other thing to be considered is that victims and perpetrators are both connected to something larger working behind them. We are being too short sighted if we only look at the victims and the perpetrators, or the living and the dead. Behind them all is something much greater that we can't identify. I call this the great soul. We are all in the care of the great soul.

To Monica You look much happier now than you did earlier. That's all.

227

HELLINGER What's the issue with the two of you?

JUSTIN We've been married for over 20 years and have two children. The early times were basically good. Over the course of time, we have moved further and further apart. At the moment, we live like brother and sister in the same house. The fire is out. I notice it in my energy level. The marriage takes too much energy. I'm always tired. I don't have the energy for sports or for my job that I used to. When I'm not in this marriage, when I'm with a woman friend, then I've got energy again and my life picks up.

HELLINGER You have a woman friend?

JUSTIN Yes.

HELLINGER For how long?

JUSTIN From time to time. At first I had a guilty conscience, but now I think it's justified.

HELLINGER Before I ask Francisca anything, choose representatives for you, your wife, and your girlfriend.

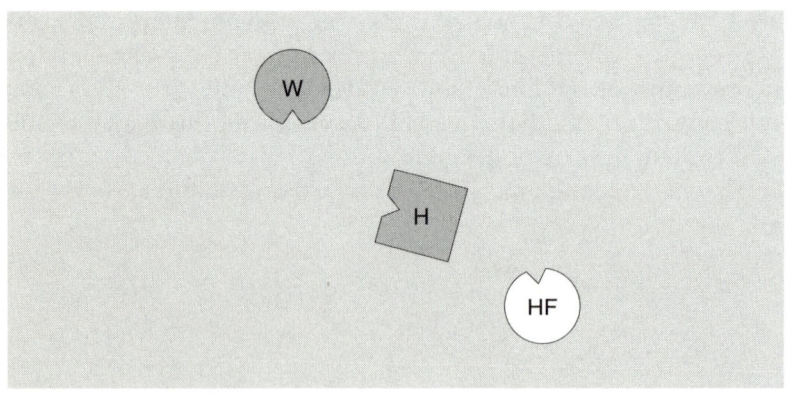

H	Husband (Justin)	HF	Husband's Woman Friend
W	Wife (Francisca)		

HELLINGER *to the representative of Francisca* How is the wife feeling?

WIFE I'd like to see the girlfriend more clearly. That is, my husband's a bit in my way.

Laughter in the group.

HELLINGER How is the man doing?
HUSBAND I feel something in my back. What I'd really like to do is just move forward and get out, but there's something holding me back. I have to keep looking over at my wife.
HELLINGER And the girlfriend?
HUSBAND'S FRIEND Pretty much the same. I'd like to take off. But I'd still like to get to know this woman, or to know who she is.
HELLINGER Go and stand next to her.

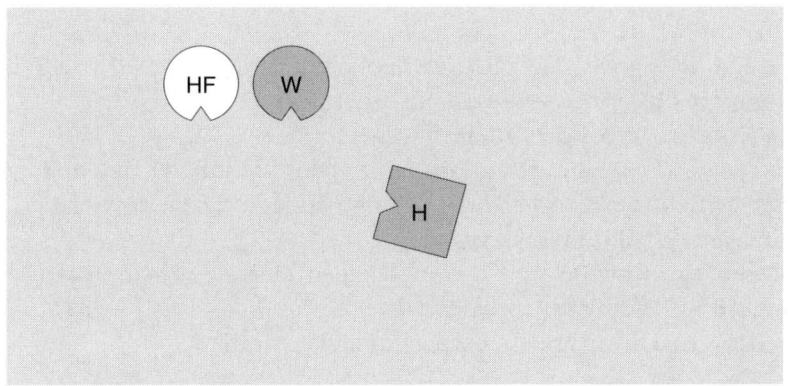

The wife laughs as the girlfriend stands next to her.

HELLINGER *to group* The wife is blossoming. It often happens that a husband's girlfriend makes his wife blossom. It's very peculiar.

The two woman laugh together.

HELLINGER *to husband's representative* How are you doing now?
HUSBAND Behind me, everything is open, and I find those two very amusing. *He laughs.*
HELLINGER Exactly.

Hellinger leads him closer to his wife.

HELLINGER Test it out, how close you want to get to her.
HUSBAND This is fine, here.

229

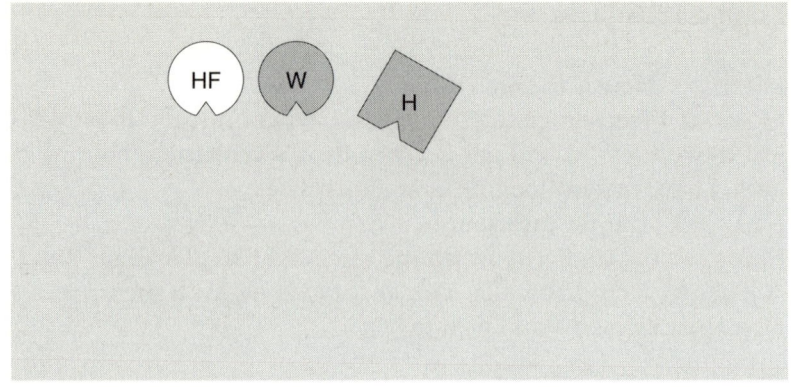

HELLINGER *to group* The girlfriend is saving the marriage, if you look at it very objectively and without any prejudices.
To Francisca What do you have to say to that?
FRANCISCA I can understand that completely. I think it's like that.
HELLINGER *to the representatives* Thank you, you can sit down again.
To Justin What do you have to say?
JUSTIN I can understand it somewhat in that the missing piece of myself is filled by my girlfriend.
HELLINGER How did you feel as you looked at that?
JUSTIN Good.
HELLINGER I'll tell you something that can help. If you've got a girlfriend, have her with respect for your wife. Okay? *Justin nods.*
HELLINGER *to Francisca* Do you want to add something more?
FRANCISCA The whole thing is a bit difficult for me, that's clear. We've had problems in our relationship for 22 years. I've never had the courage to leave, even though I wasn't happy. Somehow, we still have something to finish with each other, but I don't know what. That's why we're here, to look at what good we can bring out of it, and also for our children.
HELLINGER I'll leave it here for now. You need some time to let that have its effect on you.

230

HELLINGER *to group* In many couples, the husband imagines that he has a wife, and the wife imagines that she has a husband. The man doesn't *have* a wife and the wife doesn't *have* a husband, but rather they are two people who are brought together, through lust, through love, through hopes. These drives and hopes have a hidden agenda. Through this, the man and woman serve this goal.

After a while, the man notices that he doesn't *have* a wife, and the woman notices that she doesn't *have* a husband. At that point they let go of each other a bit and a space develops between them, as well as a bit more freedom. When the demand stops that "I *have* you and you have to *have* me", then each of them has a chance to get close to the other in a way that wasn't possible before.

HELLINGER *to Ernest and Lisa* What's going on?
LISA What's on my mind is that ever since last autumn, my husband keeps talking about death, that he can feel it, that death is very close. It frightens me. His father died a few months ago, and we lost two children. Since then I have felt a gap between us. I can't reach him very easily.
HELLINGER *to Ernest* Choose a representative for death and set up a constellation with you in relationship to death.

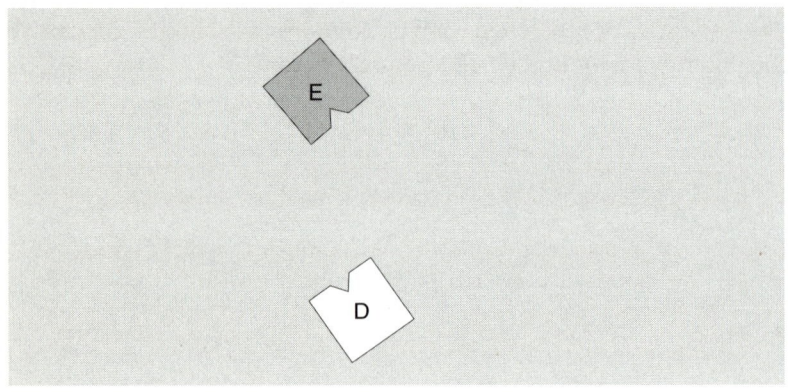

D   Death
E   Ernest

Ernest and death look at each other for a while. Then, they turn and move towards each other in tiny steps. They reach out their hands, continuing to hold eye contact.
Death lays his hand on Ernest's shoulder. Ernest lays his head on death's shoulder. They embrace with feeling. Ernest is very moved.

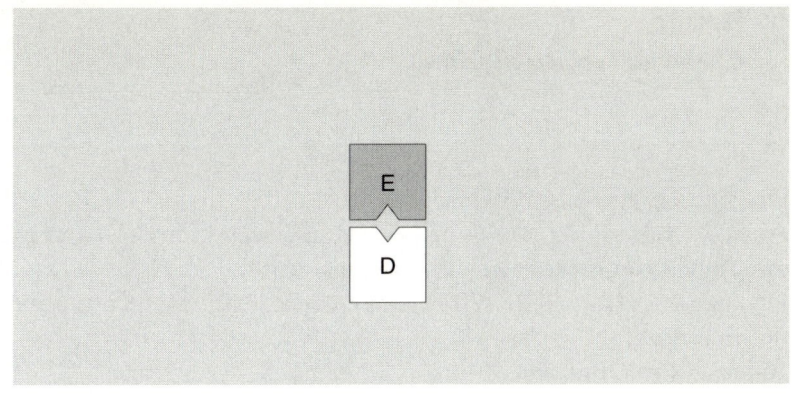

Ernest slowly frees himself from death, but they continue to hold hands and look at each other. Then, each moves slowly backwards. They stop and look at each other a while longer. Ernest turns around slowly and walks to Lisa, who is sitting next to Hellinger. He embraces her. As they release their embrace, they look at each other for a long time. He sits down next to her and they hold hands and look at each other.

HELLINGER *as Ernest and Lisa break eye contact* Okay, that's it then. All the best to you both.

Lisa smiles and nods.

HELLINGER *to Andreas* What is it?

ANDREAS I'm asking you to help me find a way to my son and my daughter. I can't take my children in my arms.

HELLINGER Are the children from this current relationship, or a previous marriage?

ANDREAS From this one.

HELLINGER Choose representatives for your children.

Andreas chooses representatives and Hellinger places them next to each other facing Andreas.

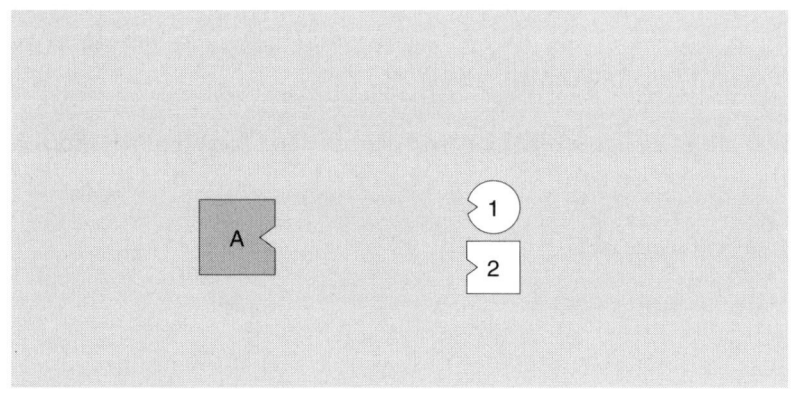

A	**Andreas**
1	First Child, a daughter
2	Second Child, a son

After a while, Hellinger chooses a representative for Andreas' father and puts him into the constellation.

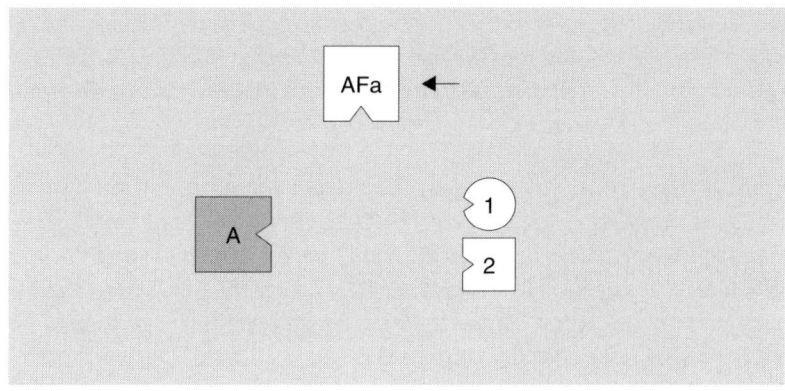

AF   Andreas' father

Andreas looks a while at his father, then at his children, and then back to his father. Hellinger turns him towards his father and they look at each other. As the father makes as though to move towards Andreas, Hellinger stops him.

HELLINGER *to Andreas* Kneel down before him and bow down all the way to the floor. Bow all the way down to the floor. Put your hands out in front of you, palms up. Put your head truly down, onto the floor.

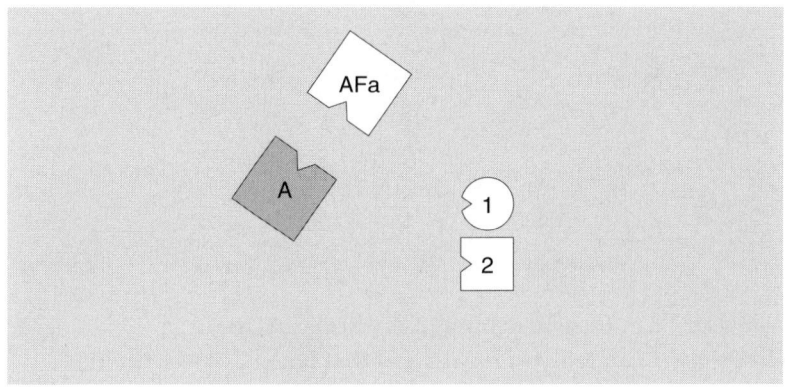

Hellinger bows Andreas' head. Andreas remains in this low bow for a long time, breathing heavily. Now and again his hands clench into fists, and then open again. His head comes up periodically, and then back down. After

235

this, he straightens up somewhat and supports himself on his hands. After a long while he bows down to the floor again, clenches his fists, then sits up again, fighting with himself. The children watch and spontaneously put an arm around each other.

Andreas wipes tears from his eyes, bows down again, then again clenches his hands into fists. Then he opens his hand and lays them flat on the floor. Finally, he straightens up, wipes the tears from his eyes, and supports himself on his arms again. He breathes deeply. During the entire time, the representative of his father stands with his hands open in front of him. The whole process takes over five minutes.

HELLINGER *to Andreas' Father* Now pull him up to you.

The father's representative bends down to Andreas, takes him by the hands, and pulls him up to him. They look each other in the eye. Andreas is still struggling with himself, but his father pulls him close. Andreas takes a while longer, but then gives in to his father and lays his head on his father's chest. He breathes deeply. Then he puts his arms around his father.

HELLINGER Now stand next to each other.

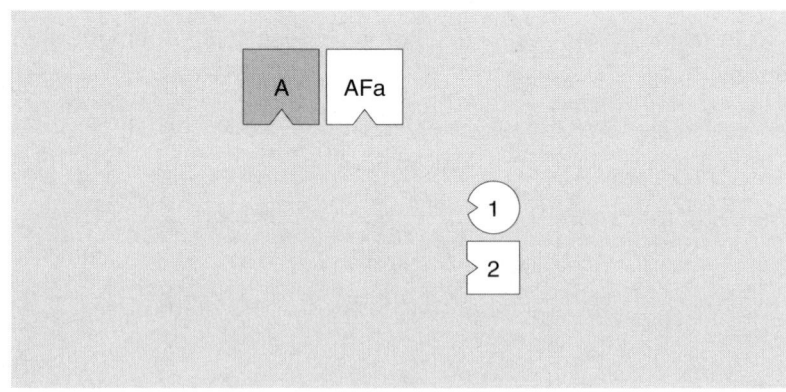

ANDREAS I can't feel anything in my arms anymore.
HELLINGER I can tell you how to get that back. Come with me.

Hellinger leads him to his son, and they embrace warmly. Cornelia, who is watching, weeps emotionally. Then Andreas also draws his daughter close to him and all three embrace.

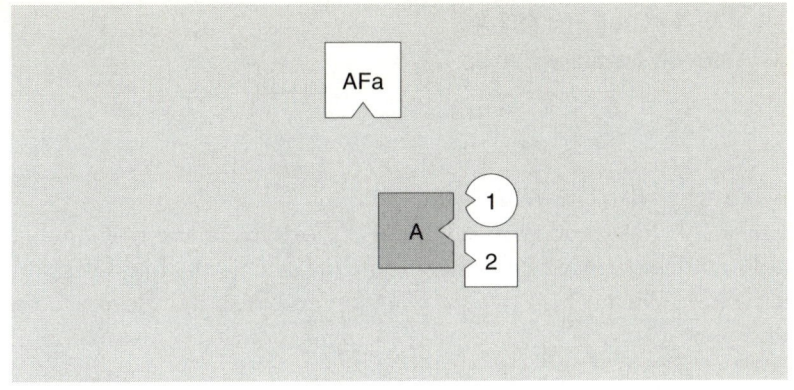

HELLINGER *to Andreas* How are you feeling now?

ANDREAS *breathing deeply* Better.

HELLINGER The daughter?

FIRST CHILD Good. Right at the beginning there was a barrier there. As soon as his father came in, he got bigger for me. As he bowed down and struggled with himself, I was proud of him.

HELLINGER *to son* And for you?

SECOND CHILD At first I was aware of my heart pounding when he stood in front of me. It touched my heart then, when he made this gesture of humility, but I had shaky knees. Things got better when he came over to us. The ground was firmer then.

HELLINGER *to Andreas* We didn't spare you anything here, thank God.

ANDREAS It's a new situation. I have to take it in first.

HELLINGER Exactly, it can grow now.

To Andreas' father's representative What was going on with you?

ANDREAS' FATHER'S REPRESENTATIVE It was very difficult not to pull him up sooner.

HELLINGER That's how fathers are. Therapists are a bit tougher. *Laughter in the group.*

Andreas and Cornelia embrace and she lays her head on his shoulder.

"I'LL BE THERE IF YOU NEED ME"
A mentally handicapped sister

HELLINGER *to Barbara* What is the issue?
BARBARA It has to do with my family of origin. I have five siblings and I'm the youngest. The sister before me is mentally handicapped.
HELLINGER We'll set up two people, you and your handicapped sister.

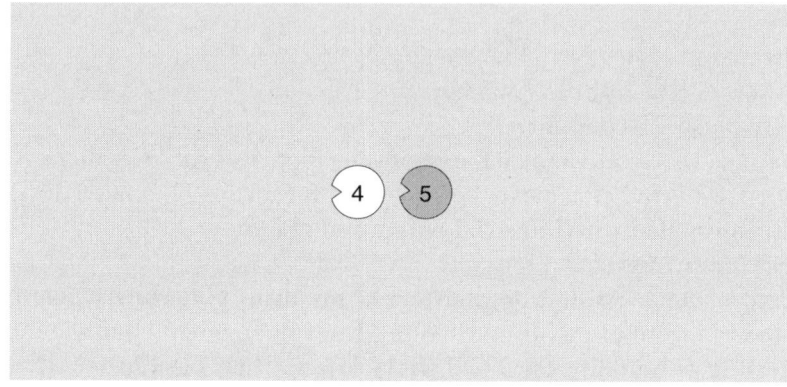

4   Fourth Child, a daughter, mentally handicapped
5   **Fifth Child, a daughter (Barbara)**

The representative of the handicapped child turns her head towards her sister and looks at her for a long time. Then she turns towards her in tiny steps and moves slightly backwards. Barbara's representative also moves a bit away. They stand facing one another. The representative of the handicapped child opens and closes her hands alternately.

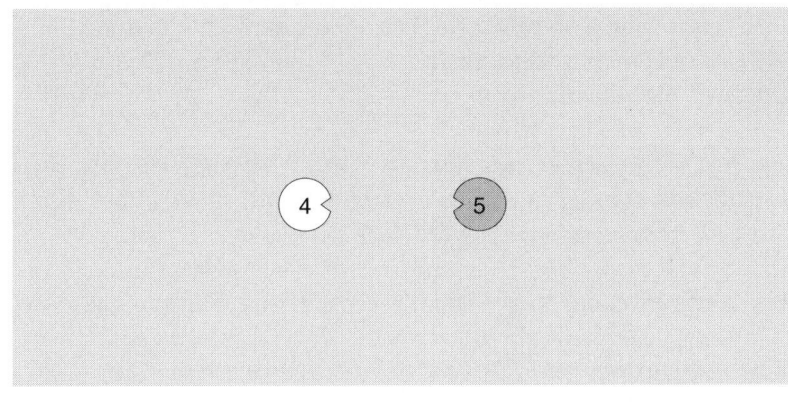

HELLINGER *after a while, to Barbara* Who does your sister live with?
BARBARA She lived with me for a few years, and now she's in a sheltered community.
HELLINGER How is she doing there?
BARBARA Not too well. She doesn't want to be there. She wants to live with me.
HELLINGER *to Barbara's representative* How are you feeling?
FIFTH CHILD I'm afraid of my sister. She's awfully powerful for me. She's challenging when she stands there.
HELLINGER *to sister's representative* What's going on with you?
FOURTH CHILD I want to keep a distance from her. I also felt afraid when we were standing so close together.
HELLINGER *to Barbara's representative* Tell her, "I am your sister."
FIFTH CHILD I am your sister.
HELLINGER "And I'm healthy."
FIFTH CHILD And I'm healthy.
HELLINGER "I take that as a special gift."
FIFTH CHILD I take that as a special gift.
HELLINGER "And I'll share that with you."
FIFTH CHILD And I'll share that with you.
HELLINGER "If you need me, I'll be there."
FIFTH CHILD If you need me, I'll be there.
HELLINGER "I'll always be your sister."
FIFTH CHILD I'll always be your sister.
HELLINGER *to sister's representative* How are you doing with that?
FOURTH CHILD I feel touched. I'm recognized for who I am.
HELLINGER *to Barbara's representative* And you?

FIFTH CHILD She is so powerful. She's more powerful than me.
HELLINGER *to sister's representative* Say to your sister, "Please."
FOURTH CHILD Please.

The two sisters look at each other for a long time and then move slowly towards each other. There are many hesitations and both show their discomfort with an opening and closing of their hands.

HELLINGER *after a while, to Barbara's representative* Risk one more step.

Both take one step closer. Barbara's representative holds out her hands to her sister. After a while they take hands and look at each other.

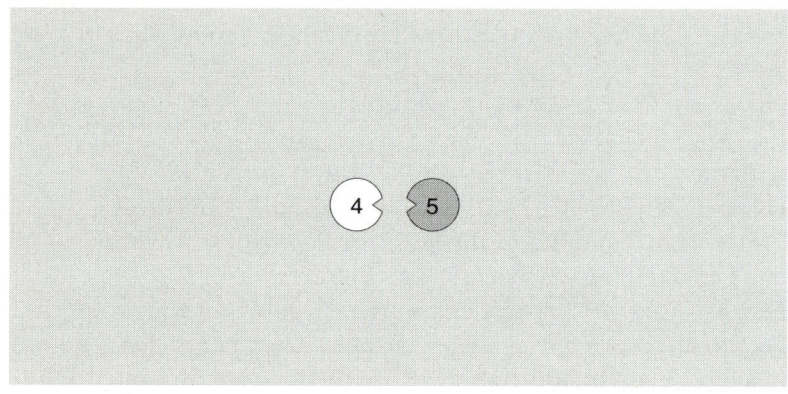

HELLINGER *to Barbara's representative* Now tell her, "Yes."
FIFTH CHILD Yes.

The sisters continue looking at each other without moving.

HELLINGER *to Barbara's representative* How are you feeling?
FIFTH CHILD I'm still a little unsure of myself. There's still something between us. I would like to get closer to her, but I am so afraid of demands, of being clawed.
HELLINGER Tell her, "I'll do anything for you."
FIFTH CHILD I'll do anything for you.
HELLINGER "Anything you need."
FIFTH CHILD Anything you need.
HELLINGER "You can rely on me completely."

240

FIFTH CHILD You can rely on me completely.
HELLINGER "I am your sister."
FIFTH CHILD I am your sister.
HELLINGER How does that feel?
FIFTH CHILD That gives me some strength.
HELLINGER Yes.
To sister's representative And for you?
FOURTH CHILD I feel very touched.

Both sisters smile and take each other in their arms.

HELLINGER *after a pause, to the sister's representatives* How is that?
FOURTH CHILD That feels good.
HELLINGER *to Barbara's representative* And you?
FIFTH CHILD I want to comfort her.
HELLINGER Good. That's it then. You've done well.

Agreeing

HELLINGER *to group* The greatness in the handicapped is astounding.
To Barbara The soul behind the handicap is great and pure. Your
representative sensed that exactly. What is required is an honoring
of the fate of the other. We've demonstrated something important
here. Often we are afraid that if we allow ourselves to get involved,
we'll be swallowed up by demands and won't have anything left for
ourselves.

I'll give you an example. There was a doctor who headed a cure
clinic for alcoholics. A former patient had phoned and asked if he
could come for therapy again. The doctor was worried that this patient would demand many sessions and he was reluctant to give him
an appointment. My suggestion was that he tell the patient, "I'll do
anything for you." He rejected that suggestion, but I encouraged him
to try it out, to see what the effect would be if he were to say that, and
really mean it. The next time I saw him, he told me that the patient
only came to see him once.

Where there is full agreement, it won't be abused. When there
are reservations, something negative creeps into the relationship that
makes both people unhappy.

This is also true for children who are worried that they will have
to take care of their parents later, and are already picturing the things

241

they will have to take on. The simple solution for this is to tell the parents, "When you need me, when you're old, I'll do anything for you – exactly the right thing." That's an important qualification.

The same is true here in relation to your sister. You tell her, "I'll do anything – exactly what is right." What is really the right thing is almost always do-able. Then you're free of the negative fantasies. Have I covered the essentials?

BARBARA Yes.

You may have been wondering about the cognitive basis that leads to the insights and resolutions that have been described in this book. My term for it is the path of phenomenological knowledge. What I mean by that, and how it differs from other paths of knowledge, is most clearly illustrated through stories.

The Recognition

There was once a man who was searching for the ultimate answer. He got on his bicycle and started off through the open countryside. Far off the beaten path, he found an unknown path.

Along this way there were no signposts, so he had to rely solely on the information he was able to obtain through his own eyes and the measure of his own steps. He was driven on by the joy of discovery, and things that had previously been premonitions now became certainties.

Finally, the path ended at a broad river and the man got off his bicycle. He could see that if he wanted to go on further, he would have to leave all his belongings on the riverbank. He would have to leave solid ground and be carried and driven on by a force much greater than himself, and he would have no choice but to entrust himself to it. The man hesitated and backed off.

As he began the ride back home, it became clear to him that he knew very little about what really helps, and he certainly couldn't pass this knowledge on to anyone else. He felt like the man on a bicycle who was following another man on a bicycle in order to tell him that his fender was loose. He shouted to the man saying, "Hey, your fender is loose!" – "What?" – "Your fender is loose!" – "I can't hear you, my fender is loose and clattering too loudly!"

The man suddenly thought to himself that something had gone wrong. So, he put on the brakes, and turned back.

A while later he met an old teacher. He asked, "What do you do when you want to help others? People often come to you to ask for advice about things you don't know very much about. But despite that, things improve for these people after talking to you."

The teacher answered, "It doesn't have to do with knowledge when someone stops and won't move forward. It's because he is looking for safety when

243

courage is called for, and wants freedom when, in fact, the correct path leaves
him no choice. And so, he goes in circles. A teacher isn't swayed by excuses
and illusions. He seeks the center and collects himself and waits – as one
who spreads the sails to catch the wind – for a word to reach him that per-
haps has an effect. When others come to him, they find him there in that
place where they themselves need to go. The answer that comes is for both.
Both are listeners."

And then, the teacher added, "And the center feels weightless."

The Scientific Way and the Path to Phenomenological Knowledge

There are two movements that can lead to insight. One is a movement that reaches out and grasps what was previously unknown,
and holds it until it is solidly owned and useable. Scientific inquiry is
a movement of this kind, and we know how much this has changed,
secured, and enriched our world and our lives.

The second movement occurs when we pause in our reaching
out, and instead of focussing on a particular, reachable object, we
look at the whole picture. Our glance can take in many things at the
same time when we allow this movement. For example, when we
look at a broad landscape or a task to be completed, or a problem to
be solved, we are aware of a view that is full and empty at the same
time. You can only see the fullness and take it in if you look away
from the particulars. In doing this, we pause in our grasping movement and pull back somewhat, until we reach an empty place that
can take in the fullness and diversity.

This pause for thought and pulling back movement is what I
would call phenomenological. It leads to a different kind of insight
than the reaching out and capturing way of knowing, and the two
complement each other. In the scientific, active way of knowing, we
have to pause sometimes to take our eyes off the narrow goal and
look at the broad picture, to look up from our close work to take in
the distance. In the reverse way, the insights gained from the path of
phenomenological knowledge need to be tested out in the particular
instance and the issue at hand.

The Process

On the path of phenomenological knowing, you surrender yourself to the multitude of particulars within a certain horizon, without choosing between them or assigning them any particular value. This path of knowledge demands an emptying of prejudices as well as an absence of inner leanings, be they emotional, intentional, or judgmental. The awareness is directed and non-directed, collected as well as empty, all at the same time.

The phenomenological attitude demands holding oneself in an alert readiness for action, but not acting. Through this tension, we are in a heightened state of awareness and readiness. Enduring this tension, you discover, after a while, that the diversity within this particular horizon connects to a center, and suddenly you see connections, perhaps even a special order of things, a truth, or perhaps the next step to be taken. This insight comes from the externals, so to speak, and is experienced as a gift. Such insight is, as a rule, limited.

Stepping Back

The first requirement for experiencing insight in this way is a lack of intention. If you have intentions, you carry your own issues into the reality, and may even change what is there to match your inner pre-formed image, and you may wish to convince or influence others according to your inner picture. If you do this, you're acting as if you are in some way superior to reality, as if the reality were the object and you the subject, instead of the other way around, with you being the object of the reality. It is clear here what is demanded of us, if we are to relinquish our intentions, even the good intentions. Quite aside from that, even common sense demands that we abandon these intentions, since our experience has shown that what is done with all good intentions, perhaps the best of intentions, very often goes wrong. Intention is no substitute for insight.

Courage

The second requirement for this kind of insight is fearlessness. If you are afraid of what reality might bring to light, you put on blinders. If you are afraid of what other people might think or do if you speak out truthfully, you narrow your vision. If a therapist is afraid to speak of a patient's reality – for example, that perhaps he does not have much more time to live – then the client will be afraid of the therapist, seeing that the therapist is not big enough to handle the reality.

Harmony
Fearlessness and relinquishing intentions enable us to be in harmony with reality, however it appears, even with those aspects which are overwhelming and frightful. The therapist is in harmony with happiness and unhappiness, innocence and guilt, health and disease, life and death. Through this harmony you gain the insight and strength to face up to the worst and sometimes, even to change it.

There's another story.

A young seeker turned to the master and said, "Please tell me what freedom is."
"Which freedom?" asked the master.
"The first freedom is foolishness. It's like the horse who, whinnying, throws its rider, only to feel the rider's grip all the more firmly the next time.

The second freedom is regret. It is like the man at the wheel who stays on board after the shipwreck instead of getting into the lifeboat.

The third freedom is insight, which comes after foolishness and regret. It is like a reed waving in the wind. Because it is so weak, it must bend, and because it bends, it remains standing."

The young seeker asked, "Is that all?"

The master added, "Some think they are seeking the truth of their own soul. But the great soul thinks and seeks through them. Just as nature, the soul can afford to make many mistakes, because she can easily replace any wrong players with new ones. However, for those who let the soul do the thinking, she sometimes allows a bit more room to move. As a river, which carries the swimmer who allows it, the soul carries this person onto the shore, using their combined strengths."

Philosophical Phenomenology
There is a difference between philosophical phenomenology and psychotherapeutic phenomenology. Philosophical phenomenology is

concerned with recognizing what is essential out of all the diversity present. If I can open myself, with every fiber of my being, what is essential appears out of the dimness like a flash of lightning. This awareness always exceeds what you could have thought up using logic, or what you might have concluded from premises or bits of knowledge, but, it is never complete. It remains enclosed in that which is inscrutable, just as everything that is, is surrounded by what is not. I can, however, grasp the essential aspects in this way. For example, it works like a systemic inner ear with a sense of balance, with whose help I can recognize immediately whether or not I am in harmony with the system. In this way I know whether that which I am doing ensures my belonging or endangers my belonging. Therefore, in this sense, a good conscience in this context means only whether I can be assured of my continued belonging to the group, and a bad conscience means only that I have to worry about not having a place in my group. This conscience has very little to do with more generally applicable laws and truths or moral judgements. It is relative and differs from group to group.

I have observed that conscience has a different role and different effects when we are talking about things that are outside the context of belonging or not belonging, as described above. A different sense of conscience comes into play within the context of the balance of giving and taking, and yet another conscience is at work that reacts to the order and hierarchy of systems. Each of these separate functions of conscience are maintained and guided by differing feelings of guilt and innocence.

The most important distinction that has been observed, however, is the difference between the conscience which is felt, and the conscience which remains hidden. What is apparent is that in following our feelings of conscience, we may violate a hidden conscience, outside our awareness. We follow our feelings, which define guilt or innocence at our level of awareness, and feel innocent in the process, but a deeper conscience deems our acts a violation and assigns guilt, with consequential effects. The opposition between these two consciences is the basis of every tragedy, which means, basically, every family tragedy. It leads to tragic entanglements with resulting accidents, severe illness, and suicide. This opposition is also responsible for many tragedies in relationships, when a couple's relationship is destroyed, despite a deep mutual love.

Psychotherapeutic Phenomenology

Psychotherapeutic insights cannot be gained through the philosophical application of phenomenology alone. Another approach is called for, which I term, knowledge through participation. This access can be opened through family constellations when conducted according to phenomenological principles.

In a family constellation, the client chooses representatives from the group of people present to represent the most important members of the family system, for example, father, mother, siblings, and the client as well. The representatives are most often unknown to the client. The client places the representatives in the space provided in relationship to one another, according to his or her collected, inner sense at that moment. Through this placement, things become apparent which may be very surprising, even to the person who has arranged the constellation. The process connects the person to a knowledge that may have been previously unavailable to him or her. For example, a colleague recently told me about a constellation in which a woman was identified with someone from the past who appeared to be a former woman friend of her father's. She asked her actual father and other relatives about this, but was assured that there was no truth in it. A few months later, her father received a letter from Belarus from a woman who had been his great love during the war. She had been trying for a long time to locate his address, and had just been successful in finding him.

The client's perspective, however, is only one aspect of this process. Another important piece of the process is that, when they are placed in a constellation, the representatives begin to have feelings which seem to be connected to the actual people they are representing, even extending to bodily symptoms in some cases. There have even been cases where a representative has heard the name of the person they were representing without the name having been spoken aloud. These experiences occur without the representatives knowing anything about the person they are representing except the position in the family and the bare external essentials. What is revealed in constellations is that a client participates in some kind of field of knowing along with other members of his or her family system and this knowledge becomes available through simple participation, without any of the usual external conduits of information. What is more surprising is that the representatives, who know almost nothing about these family members and have nothing to do with them, can connect to the reality of this family system.

This is also true for the therapists, of course. What is necessary is for the therapist, the client, and the representatives to be completely free of intent and fear, and to allow the essential reality to emerge. They have to agree to this reality as it is, without resorting to previously held theories, biases, or experiences. This is a psychotherapeutic application of a phenomenological stance. Here too, insight can only be gained by relinquishing intent and fear, and by agreeing to reality as it appears. Without this phenomenological stance, a family constellation will remain superficial and subject to error and will have little power. There has to be a willingness to agree to reality as it appears, without exaggeration or minimizing, and without any desire to interpret.

The Soul

Even more astounding than the information transmitted through participation, is the fact that this field of knowledge – I prefer to describe it as the knowing, guiding soul which transcends the individual – searches for and finds resolutions far beyond anything we could think up, and produces far-reaching effects that extend further than anything we could plan intentionally. This is clearest in constellations in which the therapist remains the least intrusive, for example, in constellations where only the most essential representatives are chosen and then left without instructions. They respond to impulses that seem to come from some irresistible force from outside themselves, which leads to experiences and insights that would be impossible in other circumstances.

Recently, during a course in Switzerland, a man mentioned, after setting up his family constellation, that he was Jewish. I set up seven representatives, standing next to one another, to represent victims of the Holocaust. I then added seven more representatives for the murderers, and had the victims face the perpetrators. The interaction between them went on for about 15 minutes without any words, and was truly unbelievable. It became clear that there was a kind of dying which remained incomplete, as well as a death that was finished. For the victims and the perpetrators, dying was completed when they could contact each other, in death, and were able to experience themselves as defined and moved and, finally, absorbed by forces with effects which extended beyond them as individuals.

Religious Phenomenology

Here, the levels of philosophy and psychotherapy are encompassed and absorbed by a greater level, at which we experience ourselves at the mercy of a greater whole that has to be acknowledged as a comprehensive finality. You could call this the religious or spiritual level. But here as well, I retain a phenomenological attitude, without intention, without fear, without pre-conceptions, and rely purely on what appears.

What that means in terms of religious insight and action is best described by another story.

The Turning Point

A man was born into his family, into his homeland, into his culture. Even as a child he was told of the teacher and master, whose example was to be followed, and he felt a deep yearning to follow this man and become like him.

He joined others who thought the same way and practiced a strict discipline for many years, following this example, until he became like the master, and thought and spoke and felt and desired like the master.

Still, he felt something was missing. So, he set out on a long journey, to seek the loneliest places and perhaps cross the last boundary. He passed by an old garden, long since abandoned, where only wild roses still bloomed, and where fruit from the huge trees fell unnoticed to the ground because there was no one who wanted it. On the other side of this garden began the desert.

Soon he was surrounded by an unknown emptiness. It seemed to him that every direction was the same, and the images which sometimes appeared before him also proved to be empty. He roamed on as he felt driven, and when he had long since given up trusting his senses, he saw a spring in front of him. It bubbled out of the earth and the water soaked quickly back into the soil. As far as the water reached, however, the desert was transformed into a paradise.

As he looked around, he saw two strangers approaching. They had done just as he himself had done, and had followed the example of their master until they were like him. They, too, had made a long journey through the loneliness of the desert in hope of crossing the final boundary. They had found, as he, the spring. All together they bent down to drink of the same water, and each believed himself to be almost at his goal. They said their names: "I am Gautama, the Buddha." – "I am called Jesus, the Christ." – "My name is Mohammed, the Prophet."

The night descended and above them, just as before, shone the stars, unreachably remote and still. They were all silent, and one of the three knew he was closer to his master than ever before. It was as if he had a sense, for an instant, of how it had been for him as he had known helplessness, futility, and humility. And how he must have felt, too, as he knew guilt.

The next morning the man turned back and escaped out of the desert. Once again he passed by the abandoned garden and continued until he came to the garden that was his own. At his gate stood an old man, as if he had been waiting for him. The old man spoke. "One who has found his way back from such a distance as you loves the moist earth. He knows that all that grows also dies, and when it is finished, it nourishes." The man answered, "Yes. I agree to the   laws of the Earth." And he began to cultivate the soil.

About the Author

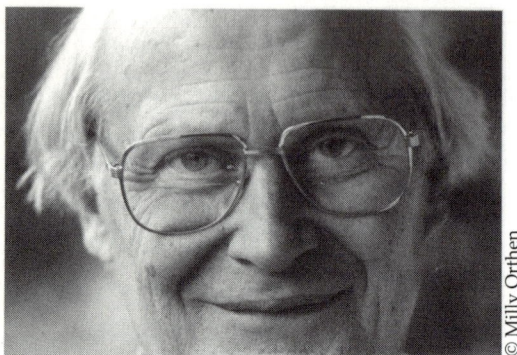

© Milly Orthen

Bert Hellinger is probably Europe's most innovative and provocative psychotherapist and a best-selling psychotherapy author. A former priest and a missionary in South Africa for 16 years, as well as an educator, a psychoanalyst, body therapist, group dynamic therapist, and family therapist, he brings a lifetime of experience and wisdom to his work. The family constellations, which have become the hallmark of Hellinger's approach, as well as his observations about systemic entaglement and resolution, have touched the lives of thousands of people and have changed how many helping professionals carry out their own work.

Publications by/about Bert Hellinger and his work

In English these books are available:

Love's Hidden Symmetry. What Makes Love Work in Relationships
Bert Hellinger/Gunthard Weber/Hunter Beaumont *1998*
    352 pages. ISBN 1-891944-00-2
    Carl-Auer-Systeme Verlag and Zeig, Tucker & Theisen, Inc.
Bert Hellinger, Gunthard Weber and Hunter Beaumont have collaborated to
present a beautiful collage of poetry, healing stories, transcripts of psychotherapeutic work and moving explanations of the hidden dynamics and symmetry love
follows in intimate relationships. Original and provocative enough to change how
you think about familiar themes.

Love's Own Truths. Bonding and Balancing in Close Relationships
Bert Hellinger/Gunthard Weber/Hunter Beaumont *1998*
    464 pages. ISBN 1-891944-48-7
    Carl-Auer-Systeme Verlag and Zeig, Tucker & Theisen, Inc.
Love's Own Truths represents another important milestone in the search toward
an even greater understanding of the intricacies of relationship and resolution.
Bert Hellinger describes „Love's Own Truths" as a fundamental statement of his
approach

Touching Love. Bert Hellinger at Work with Family Systems.
Documentation of a Three-Day-Course for Psychotherapists and
their Clients *1997*
    186 pages. ISBN 3-8967 0-022-7
    Carl-Auer-Systeme Verlag
Bert Hellinger demonstrates the Hidden Symmetry of Love operating unseen in
the lives of persons suffering with serious illness and difficult life circumstances.
This book is a full documentation of a workshop for professionals held near
London in February, 1996.

Touching Love (Volume 2).
A Teaching Seminar with Bert Hellinger and Hunter Baumont *1999*
    256 pages. ISBN 3-89670- 122-3
    Carl-Auer-Systeme Verlag and Zeig, Tucker & Theisen, Inc.
This book contains the written documentation of a three-da*y*-course for psychotherapists
and their clients. It offers mental health professionals and interested non-profes-
sional readers a look in slow-motion at Bert Hellinger and Hunter Beaumont at
work.

Acknowledging What Is. Conversations with Bert Hellinger *1999*
    162 pages. ISBN 1-891944-32-0
    Zeig, Tucker & Theisen, Inc.
Deepen your understanding of Hellinger's transformative ideas on the »Natural
Orders of Love« with his latest work - a moving dialog between the tough-minded
journalist and the »Caretaker of the Soul«.

Supporting Love. How Love works in Couple Relationships.
Bert Hellinger's Work with Couples
Edited by Johannes Neuhauser 2001
   279 pages. ISBN 1-891944-49-5
   Zeig, Tucker & Theisen, Inc.
„In this expertly edited book, Johannes Neuhauser brings an artist's eye to Bert Hellinger's unique approach, and shows that beneath the surface of his often-startling work there is a gentle tenderness that calls - softly und steadily - to the truths that lay resting in our hearts. It is refreshing in this era of psychotherapeutic relativism to come across the work of a therapist who takes a quiet and clear-sighted stand for the centrality of love in human life. The power of the work that has emerged from Hellinger's unwavering focus on the flow of love in relationships is remarkable; it will touch any who come into contact with it - professional und lay readers alike." (Arthur Roberts, M.A., Editor und Co-Director, The Gestalt Press)
The english edition of »Wie Liebe gelingt«

To the Heart of the Matter. Brief Therapies
Bert Hellinger 2002
   256 pages. ISBN 3-89670-396-X
   Carl-Auer-Systeme Verlag
Bert Hellingers's particular brand of brief therapy can be very brief indeed. Perhaps truth needn't be long-winded, just seen. Translated by Collen Beaumont.
The english edition of »Mitte und Maß. Kurztherapien«

Insights. Lectures and Stories
Bert Hellinger 2002
   138 pages. ISBN 3-89670-281-5
   Carl-Auer-Systeme Verlag
This is a first collection of Bert Hellinger's lectures and stories now translated into English. In this book he allows us to confront without fear the deep issues of guilt and conscience and brings to light the hidden orders through which love within and between people and groups succeeds. These stories attempt to lead us to a peaceful centre - a place where we can be collected and calm, in touch with our deepest love and longing, in tune with the world, and from which our relationships can be fulfilled and our lives healed. This is a book of wisdom: exciting, moving and profound.
The english edition of »Die Mitte fühlt sich leicht an«

Images of the Soul.
The Workings of the Soul in Shamanic Rituals and Family Constellations
Daan van Kampenhout 2001
   156 pages. ISBN 3-89670-231-9
   Carl-Auer-Systeme Verlag
Daan van Kampenhout and Bert Hellinger had a lengthy and intensive correspondence concerning the relation between shamanism and family constellations. The ideas explored in this correspondence formed the foundations of Images of the Soul, in which the dynamics of Hellinger´s systemic work are carefully described from the viewpoint of tradional shamanism. The book points out those spiritual principles which lie at the foundation of both shamanic practice

and family constellations, and includes many practical tips for people involved in systemic work as participant or trainer. Theoretical explorations are made concrete by examples from sessions with clients and groups, by personal experiences of the author with rituals on Indian reservations in the USA and by anecdotes from his studies with traditional medicine people and shamans.
The english edition of »Die Heilung kommt von außerhalb«

The River Never Looks Back.
Historical and Practical foundations of Bert Helinger's Family Constellations
Ursula Franke 2002
  176 pages. ISBN 3-89670-391-9
  Carl-Auer-Systeme Verlag
"The River Never Looks Back" is a book about the theory and practice of the method of systemic family constellation. Ursula Franke provides a well-grounded historical overview of the precursors to family con-stellations. In addition, she presents and defines the central termi-nology of these methods. The author presents a hypothetical model that attempts to explain the efficacy of constellations and deals with a number of questions that emerge when actually carrying them out. The empirical section of the book allows the reader to take a look at the procedure that is used in the process of a constellation, from the therapist's initial hypotheses to the resolution stage of the constellation. Franke explains, step-by-step, the application in individual therapy. In addition, the possibilities for and limitations of using constellations in individual therapy are discussed. The study presented in "The River Never Looks Back" focuses on therapy with anxiety patients. The results of the study can be used in regular psychotherapeutic practices, and is thus is helpful for all therapists who work with constellations.

The Art and Practice of Family Constellations.
Leading Family Constellations as developed by Bert Hellinger
Bertold Ulsamer 2002
  198 pages. ISBN 3-89670-398-6
  Carl-Auer-Systeme Verlag
Using the systemic family therapy developed by Bert Hellinger, tensions and conflicts within families can be revealed. Through the use of representatives, the person involved can observe the psychic dynamics of his or her own family, and identify the patterns which are destructive. In his book, Bertold Ulsamer explains the basis of family constellations, considers the task and the role of the therapist in the field of subjective experience and objective knowledge. He addresses the use of language and the issue of dealing with emotions. His book is aimed at therapists and others who are interested in the practical applications of the Hellinger therapy.
The english edition of »Das Handwerk des Familien-Stellens«

For more titles and to place your order please see:
www.carl-auer.com